Prevention
STRETCH
YOURSELF HEALTHY

Easy Routines to Relieve Pain, Boost Energy, and Feel Refreshed

DR. RACHEL TAVEL, PT, DPT, CSCS

AND THE EDITORS OF PREVENTION

Cover Photography
© Philip Friedman

Interior Photography
© Jose Luis Pelaez Inc/Getty Images: VIII; © jacoblund/Getty Images: 4; © Tom Dunkley/Getty Images 6; © PeopleImages/Getty Images: 10, 21, 38; © Tara Moore/Getty Images: 14; © jia yu/Getty Images: 18; © Amin Yusifov/Getty Images: 22-25; © Cavan Images/Getty Images: 26; © South_agency/Getty Images: 31; © Inside Creative House/iStock/Getty Images Plus: 32; © Arno Images/Getty Images: 36; © Johner Images - Plattform/Getty Images: 42; © Philip Friedman: 44-133; © Diana Davis Creative: 134

Pilates blocks by Pilates Designs
Book design by Michael Wilson
Stretches modeled by Kathryn Ross-Nash

Library of Congress Cataloging-in-Publication Data is on file with the publisher.

978-1-950099-77-1

Printed in the United States

4 6 8 10 9 7 5 paperback

HEARST

CONTENTS

FIND THE STRETCH FOR YOU

INTRODUCTION:
YOUR BODY DESERVES A STRETCH

I have a confession: I can't touch my toes. I don't think I've ever been able to—I distinctly remember being in 4th grade gym class clutching my shins while other girls had their palms flat on the floor.

Back then, my lack of flexibility didn't really slow me down: I jumped rope and ran around and did all the things a 9-year-old does. But decades later, I started to feel it. I'd go for a run in the morning and feel great, then sit at my desk for hours. When I finally got up, I'd find myself practically hobbling to the door.

When I jokingly mentioned this to a trainer I know ("Poor me, never been flexible, ha ha"), she looked at me with— well, I won't say horror, but it was close. Was I stretching, she asked? Not a lot, I told her. I don't run that fast, I protested, and honestly, I'm so busy. She gave me the kindest lecture you can imagine, which I will now summarize for you:

Your body deserves to stretch. It's the simplest and best way to feel younger, move better, and ease pain. Please do it.

How could I ignore such a plea for my well-being? I started building in a little time after my runs to stretch and getting up to loosen my muscles in the middle of my workday. My dog is a big fan of this change, since I often sit on the floor and that, of course, is an invitation for her to roll over for a belly rub.

When we started working on this book, I was delighted to get more guidance on some of my favorite stretches, but even happier to learn new ones— and, crucially, smart ways to put them together. My favorite thing is seeing how various stretches work together to prevent and relieve pain, warm up your body for exercise, or wind it down for a better night's sleep. There are so many great combinations you can try.

An amazing benefit I've discovered is in the power of taking time to pay attention to your body. I'm always rushing from one thing to the next, but by blocking out time to stretch, I'm able to find much-needed calm. It's relaxing and restorative (and I still feel like I'm being productive!).

It's been months since I got up from my desk and said "ouch." I've been running faster and enjoying every kind of movement more. I still can't touch my toes, but I'm closer than literally ever in my life—and the most important thing is this: I feel good about what my body can do. Start stretching, and I know you will too.

Sarah

Sarah Smith
Content Director,
***Prevention* magazine**

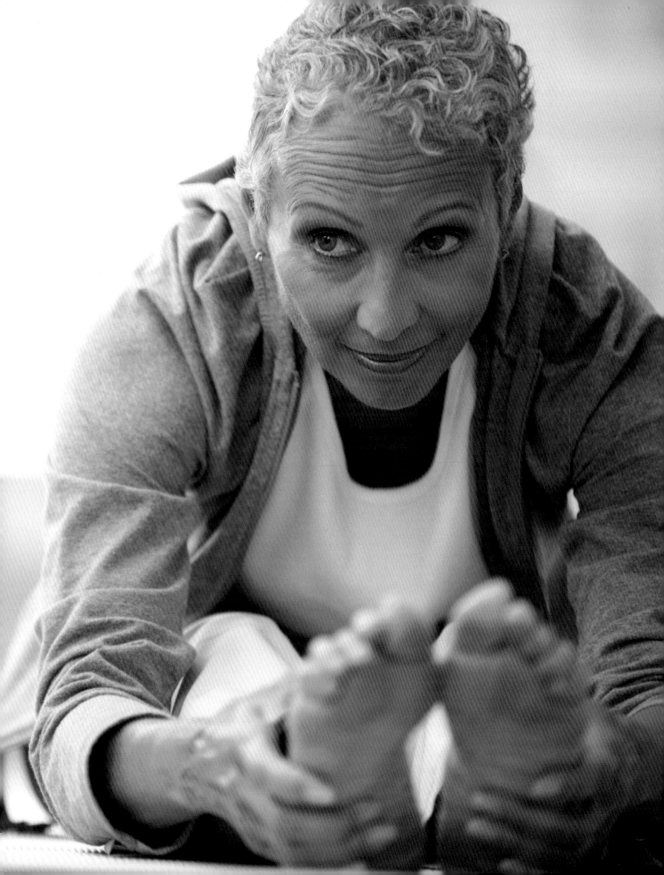

CHAPTER 1

THE POWER OF
STRETCHING

Too many of us think that to feel our best, we need to overhaul our lives. A total diet revamp, a seven-days-a-week workout routine, a commitment to 10,000 steps per day. Such weighty endeavors can be hard to stick to or even start. Sometimes just the thought of taking on such a huge lifestyle shift can seem more daunting than living with the very aches and pains we're trying to heal.

Luckily, in many cases an easier, faster, and much less intimidating approach will do the trick. If you suffer from stiff joints, tight muscles, chronic stress, low energy, and a range of other conditions, the simple act of stretching may be the answer.

Stretching has been an integral part of wellness routines around the world for centuries—and for good reason. This gentle, soothing act is one of the few physical activities that people of all ages and fitness levels can partake in. It requires nothing but your own body (and maybe the soft nudge of gravity) and can be done standing, sitting, and even lying down. You don't need any prior experience to get started. Even if you haven't logged one minute of physical activity in years, you can begin a stretching routine with ease and use it to help you achieve even some of your biggest health goals.

But before you can use stretching to tackle your wellness goals, it's worth knowing why your body could use a big stretch. Daily life requires us to have a wide range of motion, a.k.a. mobility. Twisting your neck to check your blind spot. Raising your arm to reach the top shelf at the grocery store. Bending down to pick up some boxes. Even crossing your leg to tie your shoes. These are all examples of your mobility at work. When you move in only one direction day after day or don't move your joints within their full range of motion, it can lead to limitations in mobility.

Unfortunately, modern life sets us up for these types of issues. We sit *a lot*. From in our cars on our daily commute to at our desks for hours on end, these patterns restrict our movement to a certain radius. It doesn't have to be all bad, though. Depending on the type of movement patterns in your life, they can either reinforce tightness or encourage mobility. In this book, you will learn how to increase your mobility no matter what your day-to-day activity looks like.

Moving with greater ease is one of

10

That's how many minutes of stretching it took for workers to feel lower levels of anxiety, according to a 2013 study.

the most direct benefits of adding a stretching routine to your life, but the positive impacts of this activity extend ever further. Here are some of the ways stretching can help you.

Relieves Chronic Pain

Chronic pain can enter our lives in different ways. Sometimes it creeps in slowly over the years. Other times a single event can transform our bodies in an instant. No matter the cause of your pain, you likely have one end goal in mind: Get rid of it. Too often, getting rid of pain comes in the form of expensive medications, but many types of pain can be healed by a totally different, completely free approach: stretching. According to a 2018 study in the *Journal of Complementary and Integrative Medicine,* stretching and deep-breathing exercises helped reduce pain and tension in those with neck discomfort. When performed regularly, stretching can relieve stiff muscles and soothe creaky joints from head to toe, from tight back muscles to rigid hips. Even a short session can release tension and promote relaxation.

Boosts Relaxation

Another benefit of stretching is increased relaxation. Between allowing the muscles to slowly lengthen and pairing breathwork with movement, stretching can be a very soothing experience for the mind, body, and spirit. It provides an opportunity for the mind and body to pause, be relatively still, and focus on tension reduction wherever it is felt most. In fact, research shows that stretching, when done regularly, can even boost your overall health. Doesn't that sound relaxing?

Sparks Motivation

You know how the simple act of making your bed in the morning can provide enough of a sense of accomplishment to spur you on to a totally productive day? Stretching can trigger the same sort of motivation. Studies show that even the smallest of achievements, like completing a 10-minute flexibility routine, can trigger our brain's reward circuits. This typically means a release of dopamine, the feel-good hormone. In other words, stretching is an easy win. It takes very little effort to sit on the floor, legs outstretched, and reach for your toes, but it is one important step in any fitness journey. Consider adding it to your morning routine to start the day feeling inspired.

Improves Balance

Balance is important to our lives for so many reasons. It's crucial to preventing trips and falls that can trigger injuries and makes common activities manageable, like getting up off a beach chair for instance. Luckily, you don't need to study ballet or become an expert yogi to improve your sense of balance. Elderly men who performed static leg stretches were able to balance more easily than when they did not stretch, according to a 2017 study in *The Physician and Sportsmedicine*. Even better, it took only four 15-second stretches for them to experience the boost in stability.

Improves Sleep

The relaxing effects of a good stretch can linger even after you've turned off your bedroom lights. A 2018 study in the *Brazilian Journal of Psychiatry* found that chronic insomniacs who performed resistance exercises and stretches slept better than those who did not. Try adding a couple of your favorite stretches to your bedtime routine while playing some soft music. Within a few minutes, you'll start to wind down and prepare your body for sleep.

Increases Energy

Yep, stretching has the power to lull you to sleep *or* kick-start your morning, depending on the stretches you do. Slow breathing and longer holds can be relaxing, while dynamic stretches or stretching multiple muscles in a row might be more energizing. Stretching has also been found to increase blood flow throughout your body, according to a

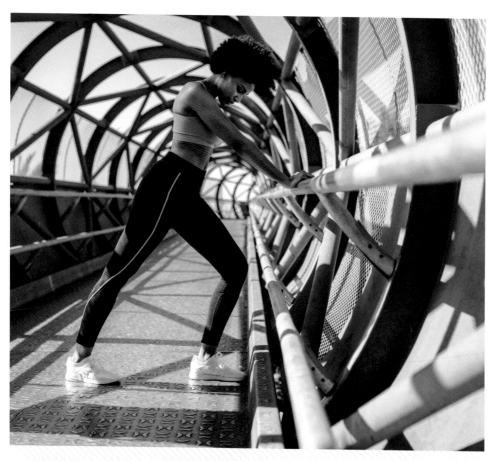

MOBILITY VS. FLEXIBILITY

Both mobility and flexibility can be improved by stretching, but they're not quite the same. Flexibility refers to how much your muscles are able to passively stretch or lengthen. Mobility refers to how fluidly and easily you actively move your joints. If you can touch your toes, you might consider yourself flexible. If you can perform complicated movement patterns, such as getting up and down from the floor without using your hands, you probably have good mobility. Ideally, you want both mobility and flexibility for healthy movement. The two often go hand and hand, but mobility does not rely only on muscle length and flexibility; it can be affected by joint health, lifestyle, and habitual movement patterns. Luckily, both can be improved with the right exercise program.

2018 study in the *Journal of Physiology*. And proper blood flow is crucial to a number of bodily functions. Increased blood flow to your muscles can help decrease muscle soreness after a workout, so you're not on the couch for three days after a visit to the gym. Better circulation also gives your brain a boost by sending more oxygen its way. Next time you're in need of a jolt, try going for some calf stretches instead of caffeine.

Decreases Injury Risk

Not only can stretching help alleviate the discomfort of existing pains, it can also help prevent new aches from arising. According to one 2015 study, a static stretching routine can reduce the incidence of injury; however, the evidence is not totally conclusive. Another scientific study found that static stretching may not be effective in preventing all injuries, but it might be minimally effective at reducing musculotendinous injuries such as tendinopathies (more commonly known as tendinitis).

Counteracts Aging

Stretching becomes particularly important as you age. That's because as you get older, natural processes occur that can affect mobility and limit flexibility. Over time, and depending on the way you've been moving and using (or not using) your body, the smooth cartilaginous surfaces where bones meet other

bones and form joints can slowly wear down (osteoarthritis), becoming more sandpaper-like than smooth. Osteophytes, or sharp extensions of bone, can form after repeated stress, leading to pain with movement. And overall joint fluidity and muscle strength and mass (as well as bone mass) can decrease, leading to further limitations in movement. With time, a lack of movement within a full range of motion that a joint allows can make it harder to achieve full mobility down the line and can negatively contribute to your overall health. Mobility (or the lack thereof) can also affect power output of muscles and lead to overuse injuries and even pain. So being "stiff" or "tight" is usually a little signal that pain could soon follow. Stretching can help prevent these restrictions from forming or address limitations as they arise.

As you can see, the power of stretching lies in its ability to tap into our mind and body. The best part? You may find that it brings you benefits beyond what we've outlined here. It's important to note that research also implicates that static stretching prior to a workout may reduce power output. So, your personal and fitness goals should be considered when deciding when and how to stretch. Ready to see what stretching can do for you? Read on for everything you need to know to get started.

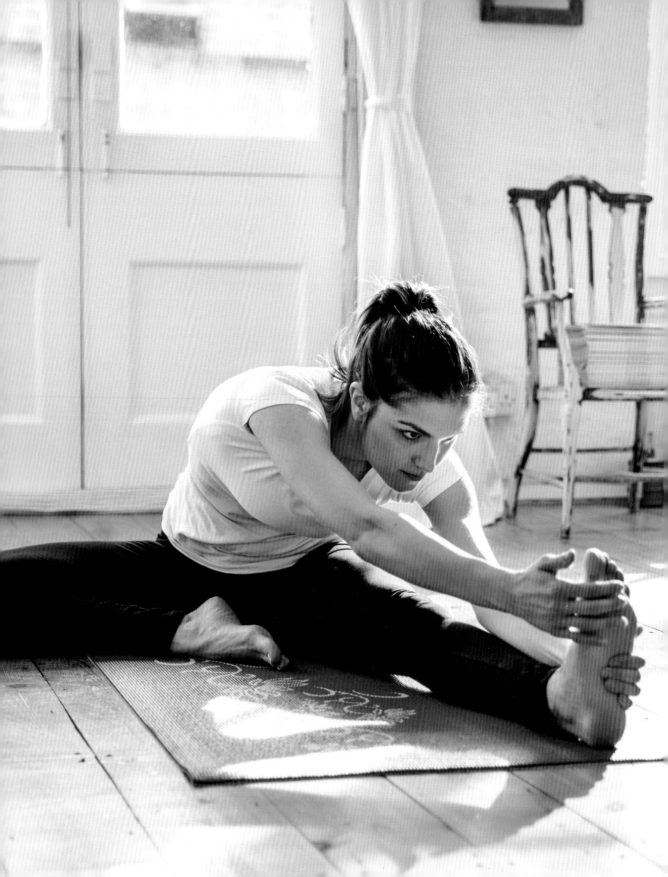

CHAPTER 2

THE BASICS OF
STRETCHING

Stretching is not complicated. It can be as simple as bending over and touching your toes. Ultimately, it's about going with how you feel and listening to your body and what it needs. However, sometimes it can be hard to interpret the signals your body is giving you. Is that pulling sensation in your neck natural or a sign it's time to stop? When you're new to stretching, every move can feel a little tight, so how can you determine what is normal and what is too much? To help you understand what a stretch should feel like so you can read your body's messages clearly, here is an overview of how this healing technique works.

What Happens to Your Body When You Stretch

There's no denying that a good stretch feels good. For some, it provides the sensation of standing a little taller or totally releasing tension. Think about how terrific it feels to stretch your arms overhead after rolling out of bed. But what's actually happening as you reach and twist and extend?

Stretching a muscle is not the same as stretching a rubber band or elastic. Unlike a rubber band, which expands and contracts in a single layer, your muscles rely on the movement of multiple layers in coordination. A whole microscopic physiologic process is taking place that includes adenosine triphosphate (ATP)—an organic compound that helps provide energy for the process—and sliding proteins. Believe it or not, the science behind understanding what actually happens during a deep stretch still has a way to go, but let's break down what we know.

First, a rundown of the many layers that exist in your muscles. Muscles are a form of connective tissue that vary in shape, size, and function, but they are all composed of the same essential parts. Striated muscles, or the type of muscles you usually think of when you imagine working out, consist of multiple strands of tissue called fascicles. These strands are further broken down into smaller bundles of muscle fibers called fasciculi. And then those bundles are made of even smaller strands called the myofibril, which is the part of the muscle that actually shortens and elongates during a stretch or a contraction. Thousands of myofibrils bundled together form each muscle fiber, and these myofibrils are composed of millions and millions of bands of sarcomeres. This is where the real action happens.

The sarcomere is the basic structural unit of muscle, where the stretching or contracting process actually takes place. Sarcomeres are composed of actin and myosin, two contractile protein filaments—the parts of your muscle that do the moving when you stretch.

So, how do these filaments actually move? The sliding filament theory helps explain it. It refers to a process believed to occur in those sarcomeres, when the muscles contract and stretch. Inside the sarcomere, it is theorized that myosin filaments slide against the actin filaments to contract or shorten a muscle. Myosin pulls itself along the actin using little extensions that look like arms reaching along a rope and hoisting itself closer. During a muscle contraction, the amount of overlap between filaments increases. When you stretch or elongate the muscles, the opposite occurs and that overlap decreases, allowing the muscles to lengthen rather than shorten.

It's not simply that a fiber gets longer or shorter. It's more about the layers of fibers and how they overlap that explains the "stretching" and "contracting" that occur when muscles are used. When a muscle is stretched or lengthened, so is a portion of it called the muscle spindle, which is a section at the end of a muscle that reports to the nervous system how quickly and how much a muscle is being stretched. When the brain senses the change is too great or too fast (or both at the same time), it signals the stretch reflex, which triggers the very same muscle you were stretching to defensively contract and go the opposite direction. This reflex is designed not to get you to spastically move but to protect your body from injury.

After a good, slow stretch, you may actually feel like your limbs are longer because you have officially bypassed the stretch reflex (the muscle spindle habituates to the new length it has achieved as its new "safe" and "normal" position) and your brain has sensed that it is safe to allow the muscles to lengthen. Many people report feeling "taller" or "longer" or "more open" after stretching. While this may actually be true due to gains in range of motion, it can also be in part to the neuromuscular system relaxing your body and letting go of some of that tension.

TYPES OF STRETCHING

Stretching can be broken down into several different categories. Although all varieties of stretching help us achieve the ultimate goal of loosening our muscles, some types are better suited than others for specific needs. Here's what you need to know:

Dynamic Stretching

Dynamic stretching is performed while moving, often mimicking movements of the sport or activity that you plan to perform. It often factors in explosive movements such as sprinting, jumping, or cutting. Because of all this movement, dynamic stretching creates more heat in the body and can better prepare you for rigorous, fast-paced activity. Think of swimmers before a race. They often perform dynamic stretches, swinging their arms around to promote mobility and readiness in their joints. Dynamic stretching in particular appears to help in warming up the muscles, which makes the joints more mobile, the tendons more compliant, and the body more prepared to perform a specific activity.

With dynamic stretching, it's always good to target the primary muscle groups you plan to use. For most people, this means the larger muscle groups of the lower extremities, such as the hamstrings, quadriceps, and glutes. The smaller workhorse muscles such as the gastrocnemius, the muscle that creates the bulging shape in your calf, and soleus, located right below it, are also extremely important to activate, as they help generate power and propulsion in sports such as running, basketball, and football.

EXAMPLES OF DYNAMIC STRETCHES:

- Leg Swings (p. 127)
- Arm Swings (p. 120)
- Butt Kicks (p. 122)
- High Knees (p. 125)
- Frankensteins (p. 124)
- Walking Lunges (p. 132)
- Squats (p. 131)
- Skipping (p. 130)
- Side Shuffles (p. 129)
- Jumping Jacks (p. 126)

Static Stretching

Static stretching is performed in a stationary position, with a sustained hold in a position that lengthens a certain muscle. You'll usually spend at least 30 seconds in a static stretch. Many yoga positions are examples of static stretches—think about holding downward dog for half a minute. According to some research, static stretching can actually have an inhibitory effect on muscle power. In other words, by lengthening the muscles and holding them in that position for an extended period of time, the muscles appear to conjure less force when tested by resistance training afterward. That leads some to argue that static stretching can have a negative impact on performance. However, its ability to gradually ease

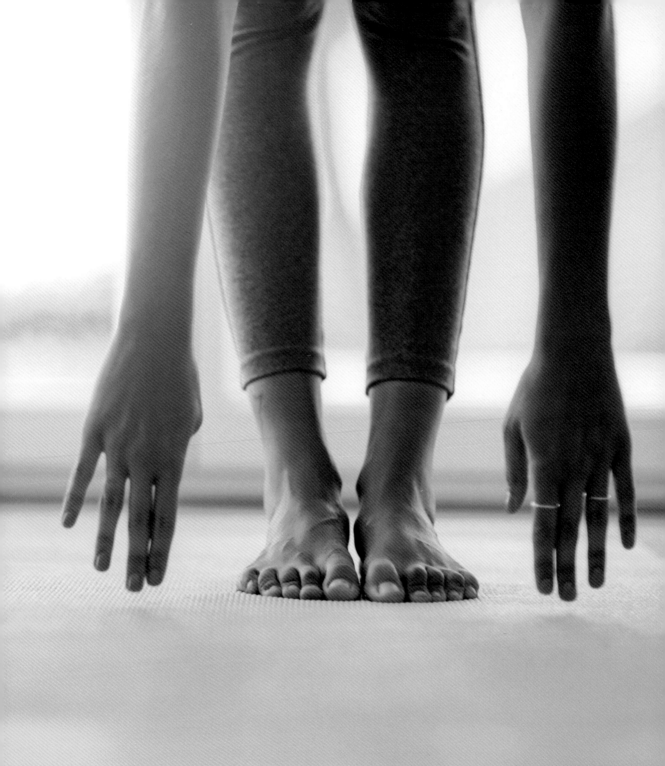

HOW IS YOUR MOBILITY?

It can be a little trickier to measure how mobile you are versus how flexible. Answer these questions to get an idea of your current range of motion.

1. **Turn your head all the way to the right. How does it feel?**
   a. Totally pain-free.
   b. Fine, until I get about 75% of the way.
   c. Tight, it's easier to turn my whole body!

2. **While standing, slowly reach down to touch your toes. How far can you go without bending your knees?**
   a. All the way to the floor.
   b. Halfway (touching knees but keeping legs straight).
   c. It's too uncomfortable. I have to bend my knees to roll down!

3. **Try to squat, lowering yourself until your butt touches the ground and both knees are totally bent.**
   a. Easy, what now?
   b. I can get about halfway before things get hard.
   c. You want me to do what?! Not even going to try!

MOSTLY A'S: VERY MOBILE

You seem to be quite flexible and comfortable with movement. Keep up the awesome work! In order to stay mobile, continue your regular stretching routine, and maintain an active lifestyle that encourages your body to move in all different ways.

MOSTLY B'S: COULD USE WORK

You're at a great place to start a stretching routine. Seems like you have some mobility and movement, but there is room for progress. No problem! Begin your weekly stretching routine, and retake this quiz in a few weeks. You're likely just a few stretches away from noticing improvement. While you might not be the most flexible person in every room, you have enough mobility to have healthy movement patterns. Begin stretching to take your mobility and flexibility to a new level.

MOSTLY C'S: NEEDS IMPROVEMENT

Sounds like you could use this book! If you want to move pain-free down the road, now is a good time to get started with some of the large-muscle basic stretches outlined in this book. But don't fret: It's never too late to start stretching and make improvements. Your future body will thank you.

your body into a position makes it ideal for increasing flexibility and promoting rehabilitation after an injury.

Static stretching can be further broken down into:

Active stretches—you do the work to increase the intensity of your stretch

Passive stretches— another individual or a tool does the work to increase the intensity of your stretch

EXAMPLES OF STATIC STRETCHES:
- Any Hamstring Stretch (p. 108)
- Lunge Stretch with Overhead Reach (p. 101)
- Calf Stretch (p. 105)
- Pec Stretch (p. 92)
- Knee to Chest Stretch (p. 95)
- Child's Pose (p. 81)
- Upper Trap Stretch (p. 117)
- Wrist Stretch (p. 77)

Ballistic Stretching

Whether at the gym or on television, you've likely seen someone perform some enthusiastic ballistic stretching before. This controversial method involves bouncing in and out of a stretch in order to create momentum and deepen the extension. For example, you might bend over and touch your toes then begin to bob your upper body up and down. This is a ballistic stretch. Researchers have warned against the use of such jerky movements as they have been shown to cause injuries by sparking your stretch reflex, which is your body's response to entering too deeply into a stretch too quickly. We haven't included any ballistic stretches in this book because they can be too dangerous to do without supervision.

PICKING THE RIGHT STRETCH

Finding the perfect stretch for your needs doesn't have to be complicated. First, ask yourself: Why are you stretching? Is it to relieve pain in specific areas? Is it to prevent injury during a workout? Is it to become as flexible as you were when you were 10? You might find that you have more than one reason, and that's okay. As you progress in your stretching routine, you might even discover that your needs evolve. What first started as a ritual to reduce pain may inspire you to set a goal of touching your toes without bending your knees. Whatever your intention, knowing the primary uses for dynamic and static stretches can help you choose the perfect stretch every time.

When to Use Dynamic Stretches

More and more evidence favors dynamic stretching over static stretching to help prevent injuries and loosen tight muscles. It may even help enhance athletic performance, which makes it especially useful before playing a sport, like basketball or baseball. One study found that dynamic stretching, with or without the addition of static stretching, was effective at improving sprint times in runners.

So, what does this mean for you? While this study applies to athletes, the science works for nonathletes as well. Anyone who engages in some type of physical activity, whether a jog or a power walk, can benefit from dynamic stretching because it can help improve range of motion and flexibility at a joint, two things you need for any kind of successful movement. Everyone has a "normal" range of motion in which they operate. Your range depends on multiple factors, including athleticism, age, and activity level. The key to dynamic stretching is that you push your body just a little outside of that typical range of motion in order to prepare for the full-blown dynamic movements you're about to perform, like in a HIIT workout or a Tabata training session.

Even while the research can't promise that dynamic stretching will prevent injury, it does seem to be effective at improving performance without doing any harm. Ultimately, dynamic stretching is most effective and productive when it comes to achieving gains in sport-specific movements or in promoting blood flow to the muscles prior to activity.

When to Use Static Stretches

That said, sometimes a static stretch can better serve you. When you have significant deficits in flexibility—say you are recovering from an injury or are post-op after a surgery—you definitely want to work on static stretching before introducing dynamic stretching to your routine. The body needs a certain baseline of muscle length and mobility to be able to effectively dynamically stretch and prevent both injury and the stretch reflex from (literally) kicking in. Static stretching also makes more sense for people performing slower movements than those needed for a game of tennis, for example. If walking is your go-to workout and you don't plan on doing any big, fast movements that reach the endpoints of your flexibility at each joint, then static stretching is great. And if flexibility in general is your main goal, this slow and gradual method can help you safely limber up.

WHAT TO DO AS YOU STRETCH

Now that you understand how to choose the perfect stretching style for your needs, you can start to think about how to actually perform it. One of the great things about stretching is that there isn't much to actually *do* as you do it. It's more about letting your mind and body relax. However, there are some best practices to be aware of to ensure you get the best stretch possible and avoid injuring yourself. Before starting any stretch, be sure to read through the instructions for how to settle into it (in chapter 8). This will help you get familiar with how your body should be aligned during a stretch and where you should feel the stretch most. Once you're

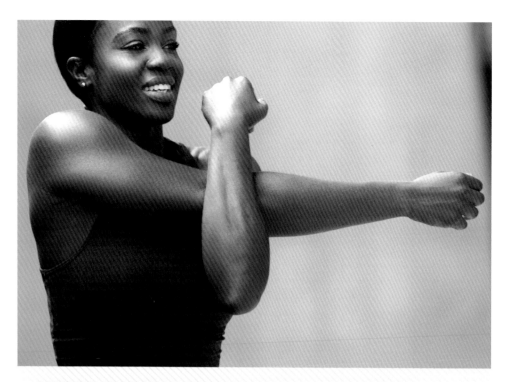

AVOID THESE 3 STRETCHING MISTAKES

1| LOCKING YOUR JOINTS

Stretching with your joints in a locked, or super straight, position can actually cause pain and stiffness. Leave a little bend to protect your cartilage. And P.S.: Don't worry if you can't touch your toes without bending your knees yet. You can gradually work toward fully extending them.

2| CUTTING IT SHORT

To see a benefit from any type of stretch, you should hold it for at least 30 seconds. Some stretching styles even call for holding a stretch for as long as 5 minutes.

3| BOUNCING AND BOBBING

Fast, jerky bouncing movements during a stretch can actually cause injuries by pushing you beyond your stretching threshold. Instead, gradually ease into a position and remain mindful of how you're feeling every inch of the way.

in the position, keep in mind the tips in the following section to help you get the most out of any stretch you're in.

How Long to Hold a Stretch

The amount of time you need to spend in a particular stretch and in your stretching routine overall depends on a range of factors. These include the type of stretch you're doing, your general mobility and comfort with movement, the type of activity you will be performing after stretching, and the amount of muscles you intend to stretch. Will you be stretching one body part in particular? Or will you be doing a full-body stretching routine? According to research, the greatest improvement in range of motion occurs after 2 to 4 repetitions of 10 to 30 seconds of static hold stretching. That said, some people might feel it takes longer to relax and ease into the stretch. Stretching requires the body to relax, and sometimes the brain can get in the way of that. So, the key is to feel the stretch not just time it. Take a deep breath, exhale, and allow your body to unwind. If you're holding a stretch for 30 seconds but you haven't actually allowed the stretch to happen, you will likely feel the same way as when you started, and the stretch will not be effective.

Actually letting yourself be fully immersed in a stretch can be easier said than done. Take a moment now to try for yourself. Stand up. While standing, slowly allow your head to tilt forward as you tuck your chin toward your chest.

Think about your spine as a long chain of beads, and allow the beads at the top to slowly fold over one bead at a time as you allow your head and shoulders to lower toward the floor. Keep your knees straight, with a slight softness behind them to prevent pain. Continue to fold over and lower your hands toward the floor, letting your head and neck release as you begin to feel a pull in the back of your legs. While bent over, take a deep breath; as you exhale, allow yourself to fall deeper into this stretch. Hold this position. See if after 10 seconds you can go just a little farther. After 30 seconds, return to standing upright by reversing the roll-up through each bead from the bottom up. Take a couple breaths before trying the stretch again. Notice how your hands might get slightly farther each time.

Each stretch—especially those targeting larger muscle groups such as the hamstrings and quadriceps—should be held for at least 30 seconds to achieve the full benefits. If you are focusing on one muscle group or body area, you will want to perform each specific stretch 2 or 3 times. For a full-body stretching routine that targets multiple muscle groups, you could spend as long as half an hour or more stretching. How long you spend on your stretching routine depends on your goals and personal preference.

What a Stretch Should Feel Like

This is one of the most common areas of

confusion for those new to stretching, and it's totally understandable. The stretching "sweet spot," generally speaking, should be somewhere between slightly uncomfortable but not painful. It should feel like a pulling sensation in the tissue but not a sharp, pointed pain. A stretch should gradually feel a little more comfortable with time and breathing, reducing tension as you allow your body to relax into it. You'll want to ease into a stretch and take it slow, breathing as you allow the muscle to lengthen. Nothing should feel forced or aggressive. It should eventually feel good, like a change is happening while you do it.

Stretching should not be done quickly or suddenly as this can trigger the body to react by slamming on the brakes as if a joint is out of control. While stretching is often not the most comfortable sensation—especially in our tightest and most limited areas (where we need it most)—a taut pulling sensation like a rope is being stretched out is okay. But don't go past that point; a sharp or painful sensation means you may be overstretching the tissue, which can lead to damage and potential inflammation rather than allowing the gentle lengthening of the tissue to occur.

How to Breathe During a Stretch

If you've ever tried to stretch a tight muscle while holding your breath, you may notice it's not easy. The way you breathe while stretching should match the desired process. To energize and activate your system, quick shallow breaths send signals to your brain that you want to move. If you are performing a static stretch, you'll want to take slow, deep diaphragmatic breaths, allowing yourself to sink deeper into the stretch on every exhale.

Diaphragmatic breathing (or abdominal breathing) is a technique used to increase the exchange of oxygen and carbon dioxide in the body and calm the nervous system by lowering the heart rate. It is used often in yoga and other practices and promotes control of the primary respiratory muscles such as the diaphragm.

Exhaling while you sink into a stretch allows the parasympathetic nervous system to activate, encouraging the "rest-and-digest" (vs. "fight-or-flight") response to occur. This promotes calm and relaxation in the body. By controlling your breathing, you can actually affect the response of your muscles.

Signs You're Overstretching

There is a fine line between your personal stretching limit and the point of overstretching. After all, a good stretch should be slightly uncomfortable, so how do you know when you've pushed it too far? You'll know you're overdoing it if you feel sharp pain or intense discomfort. Inch away from that point a little and see if you can maintain a slightly less intense stretch. Also, check your body positioning to make sure that the area where you are feeling the stretch is the area you intend to stretch. If you're feeling it at another body part, you may be compensating by pushing yourself into a stretch from the wrong place.

Another sign you've overstretched is if you activate the stretch reflex. When a muscle is stretched, this also stretches something called the muscle spindle—a section of the muscle that senses proprioception, or nerve endings in the body that relay crucial information about the musculoskeletal system to the central nervous system. These receptors tell your brain when there is a change that can be harmful to the body, among other things. The stretch reflex is a reaction designed to protect your muscles from tearing or overstretching. The quicker these proprioceptors sense a sudden change in the length of the muscle, the more quickly this reflex kicks in to recoil the muscle and prevent it from further stretching. This is part of the reason you want to hold a static stretch and ease into it slowly. By going slowly, you can bypass that stretch reflex and feel more confident that you are not overstretching.

How to Heal an Overstretched Body Part

It is possible to misread your body's warning signs and overstretch in the moment, but the consequences will be pretty clear by the next day. If you feel sore the day after stretching, it could mean you overdid it. That's because overstretching can cause tears in your muscle tissue. But this doesn't have to mark the end of your stretching journey. If you have overstretched a body part, either from stretching or from activity that has caused an injury, you'll need to take care of it so that it can heal properly. Overstretching can lead to a muscle strain, which—like most injuries—can come in varying degrees of severity. Symptoms of a strain include pain, soreness, stiffness, limitations in mobility, and even swelling or bruising. Your muscle may feel weak or limited as a result. If you suspect a strain or overstretched muscle, start by icing it, resting it, and potentially seeing a doctor or physical therapist to assess the damage and get a proper treatment plan. Very gentle stretching might be a part of the rehabilitation process, but it is important to know how injured the tissue is before doing this.

If you feel you have overstretched a body part while performing a static stretch, take a break from the stretching, and try moving normally to determine if it is a temporary sensation or an injury that may have longer-lasting effects. Healing overstretched tissue requires time and the proper protocol to reduce inflammation, maintain range of motion, and improve strength without causing pain.

Now that you know the basics of stretching, the real fun begins! In the next chapters, we'll show you how to create a stretching routine that fits your life, living space, and needs.

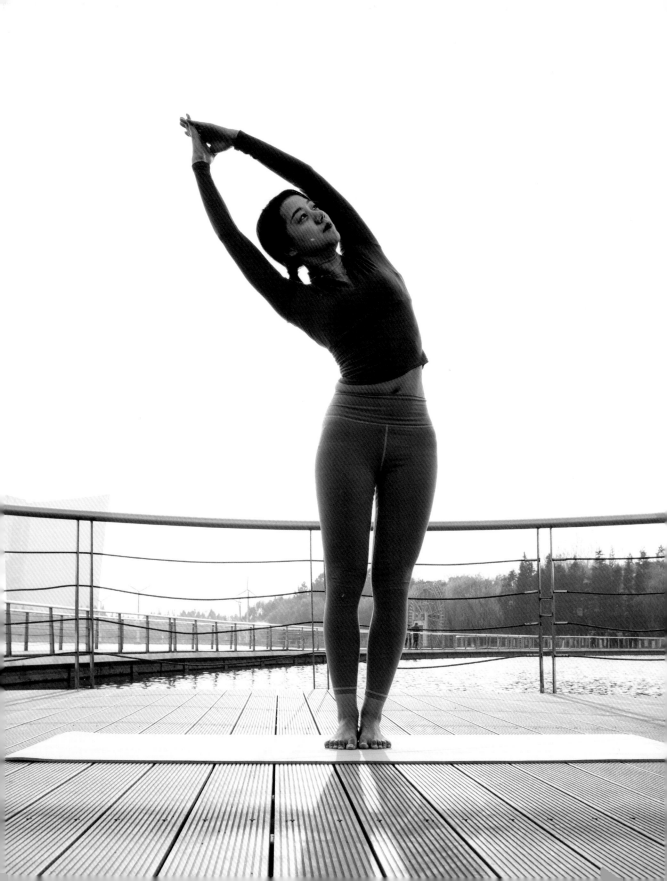

CHAPTER 3

WHAT TO STRETCH **WHEN**

There are more than 600 muscles in your body. You won't be able to give every single one a little T.L.C. every time you stretch, so it's important to know which body parts to prioritize and when to give them your full attention.

When it comes to the human body, you might think of it as separate parts. Your arms are different from your neck, which is different from your ankles. But it's important to keep in mind that everything is connected. While the connection from one body part to another might not necessarily mean they are touching (e.g., a muscle in your neck is not directly attached to a muscle in your lower leg), our muscles and body parts do not operate in isolation. In fact, the body is an amazing balancing act of coordination, weight shifting, and balance that allows us to shift from side to side as we move. While this is happen-ing, different body parts must work together to both create power and movement and stabilize the body. One part of the body can easily affect another part, and if there is tightness or dysfunc-tion in one area, you bet this could neg-atively impact another area. So how does this relate to stretching?

As far as identifying what muscle to stretch and when, most people use pain or tightness as a guide. If an area feels tight, they will try to isolate and stretch that muscle group. For example, if the calf feels tight, you might feel compelled to do some lunges or calf stretches off a step. If your lower back has pain, you might home in on that specific area by foam rolling or massaging it.

While this is not wrong, it is not the most effective and complete way of approaching stretching. Because of the interconnectedness of the body and tissue such as fascia that encapsulates all the muscles and creates connections at different levels of the body, it is important to think of stretching more broadly than we usually do.

For best results, stretch not just the primary area of concern (such as the calf muscles) but also the muscles above and below that area. Often, when one muscle is tight, other muscles along that "chain" or line are also tight. For example, consider the gastrocnemius, the large muscle that creates the bulging shape in your calf. In this case, the hamstrings or the hips may also be tight, contributing to a pull that is felt in the calf. But this tension goes up and down the chain. Where the gastrocnemius muscle starts, the hamstrings end, crossing behind the knee and potentially limiting range of motion at the knee or elsewhere.

Your best bet is to incorporate a full-body stretching routine to address all the interconnected parts. Believe it or not, right shoulder tension can also be connected to left hip tightness and so on. Zoom out on the body instead of solely homing in on the area where pain or tension is felt, and you are more likely to avoid chronic pain or acute injuries.

The following is a list of some of the most common areas of pain. As always, pain doesn't have a one-size-fits-all treatment. If you are experiencing pain, notify your doctor or physical therapist for a complete, individualized assessment and personalized treatment plan. That said, if you are experiencing some tightness in one of the areas mentioned on the next few pages, you can begin by trying to stretch it and the surrounding areas.

DID YOU KNOW?

You use most of your muscles throughout every day whether you intend to use them or not. Sometimes it's obvious—like when you get out of bed or take the stairs. Other times, like when you're standing still, you might not even realize all the muscles at work. Even sitting requires some muscle!

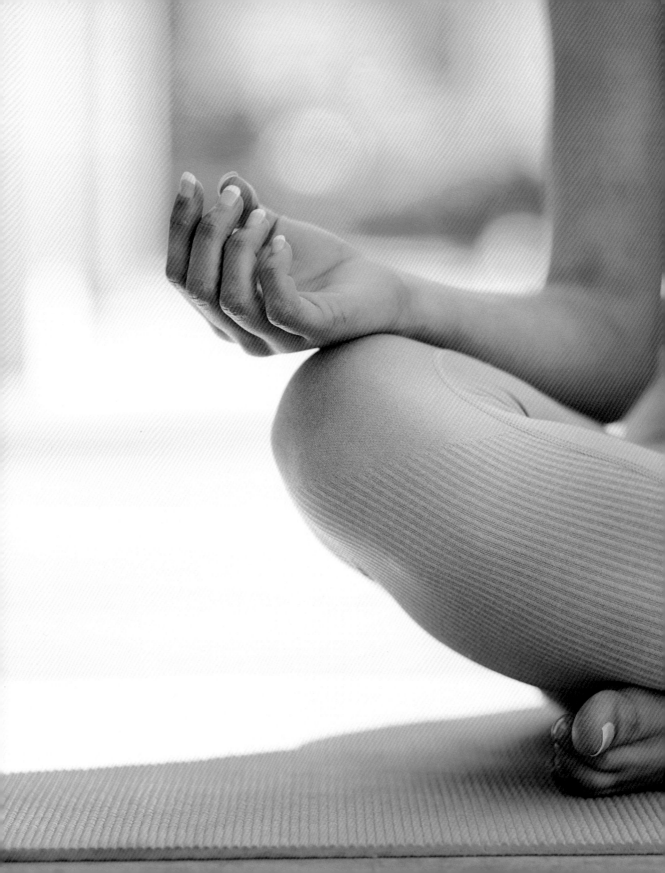

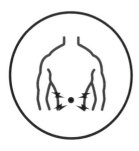

Lower Back Pain

Lower back pain is the most common area of pain. Usually it takes a multi-pronged approach to treat this type of pain, as it can be difficult to stretch the exact area of tension or pain. Working on spinal mobility and stretching some of the large surrounding muscles are usually good ways to start. Exercises such as cat-camel, lower trunk rotation, and gentle side bends can help mobilize the vertebrae. The back is central in our body and is the area from which all the extremities extend outward. This means that it is literally connected to all our other parts, including being more directly connected to the shoulders and pelvis. With this in mind, if you are experiencing low back pain, it is important to also stretch connecting musculature such as the glutes and hamstrings, as well as the pecs and muscles of the anterior hip. Tension in any of these areas can contribute to limitations in mobility leading to pain and stiffness in the lower back.

STRETCHES TO TRY:
- Cat-Camel (p. 79)
- Lower Trunk Rotation (p. 84)
- Any Hamstring Stretch (p. 108)
- Hip Stretch Off Elevated Surface (p. 102)

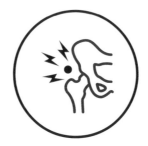

Hip Pain

If you are experiencing hip pain or tightness, remember that there are many muscles to address in the hips, depending on the specific type of pain. You'll want to stretch not just the muscles on the front, side, and back of the hips but also some of the large muscles of the legs, including the quads and hamstrings, and work on spinal mobility, since the lower back connects directly to the pelvis.

STRETCHES TO TRY:
- Figure Four Stretch (p. 96)
- Hip Stretch Off Elevated Surface (p. 102)
- Kneeling Lunge Stretch with Bent Knee (p. 100)
- Knee to Chest Stretch (p. 95)

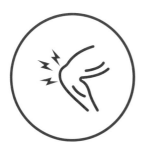

Knee Pain

Knee pain is a little more specific than hip or lower back pain. While stretching other parts of the body may provide some relief, you'll want to start by focusing on the muscles directly surrounding the knee, such as the hamstring, gastrocnemius, and quadriceps. If pain and stiffness are not relieved by stretching these muscles, look at the joints above and below the exact area of pain; these may be contributing to your pain. For example, ankle stiffness and hip weakness can lead to pain in the knee as can structural problems in the joint and will need to be assessed more carefully (stretching isn't always the solution to pain). But you can start with these stretches targeting the major muscles of the leg and go from there.

STRETCHES TO TRY:
- Quad Stretch (p. 113)
- Any Hamstring Stretch (p. 108)
- IT Band "Stretch" (p. 99)
- Calf Stretch (p. 105)

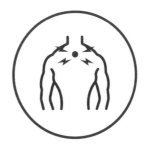

Upper Back Pain

Unfortunately, this type of pain is quite common, particularly in anyone who spends several hours working at a computer or desk (which is almost all of us!) or on the phone, as well as in upper body athletes and even parents of little ones. The upper back is connected with the lower back, neck, and shoulders. You'll want to address muscles in all these areas for a more complete stretching routine, with particular focus on the pectoralis muscles, which tend to get tight with forward body postures, limiting extension and mobility in the upper back.

STRETCHES TO TRY:
- Cat-Camel (p. 79)
- Any Pec Stretch (p. 92)
- Upper Trap Stretch (p. 117)
- Lying-Down Thoracic Extension Stretch (p. 91)

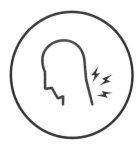

Neck Pain

Pain in your neck is often triggered by repeated phone or computer use. While this body part might seem small compared to many others, it can be quite uncomfortable to have pain or stiffness in this area. The neck, like the back, is actually very interconnected with the rest of the body through the nervous system. Neck pain should definitely be assessed by a medical professional before self-treating. General neck stiffness and tightness can be addressed with some gentle spinal mobility exercises and stretches that target the shoulders, chest, upper back, and neck muscles directly.

STRETCHES TO TRY:
- Upper Trap Stretch (p. 117)
- Any Pec Stretch (p. 92)
- Levator Scap Stretch (p. 116)
- Neck Extension over
  Foam Roller (p. 115)

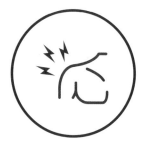

Shoulder Pain

Shoulder pain is quite common and often linked to pain in other places, from the neck and upper back to the low back or even hip. A safe place to start is usually stretching the chest muscles, neck, arms, and upper back. This might sound like a lot, but it's all directly connected to the shoulders, and tension in any of these places can affect posture, contributing to limitations in mobility in a notoriously finicky joint.

STRETCHES TO TRY:
- Any Pec Stretch (p. 92)
- Biceps Stretch (p. 76)
- Child's Pose (p. 81)
- Cat-Camel (p. 79)

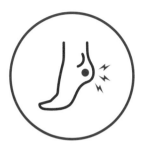

Heel Pain

Heel pain is common in runners as well as people who wear flat, hard footwear for work. It is usually associated with plantar fasciitis—an inflammation of the plantar fascia at its attachment point to the calcaneus, or heel bone. While most people think to address this type of pain by rolling out the plantar fascia itself, which can feel temporarily relieving, this type of tension and pain usually develops from tension and tightness originating higher up in the calf and leg. Be sure to stretch the hamstrings, gastrocnemius, soleus, and big toe muscles (yes, don't forget the big toe!) for a more thorough and effective stretching approach.

STRETCHES TO TRY:
- Calf Stretch (p. 105)
- Soleus Stretch (p. 112)
- Any Hamstring Stretch (p. 108)
- Big Toe Stretch (p. 104)

DON'T FORGET TO BREATHE

No matter what type of aches and pains you're experiencing, deep, slow breathing can help bring relief. As you enter a stretch, inhale for 8 seconds. Inch a little farther into the position and exhale for 8 seconds. This will help you move through your body's stretch reflex, which is telling you "Do not pass go."

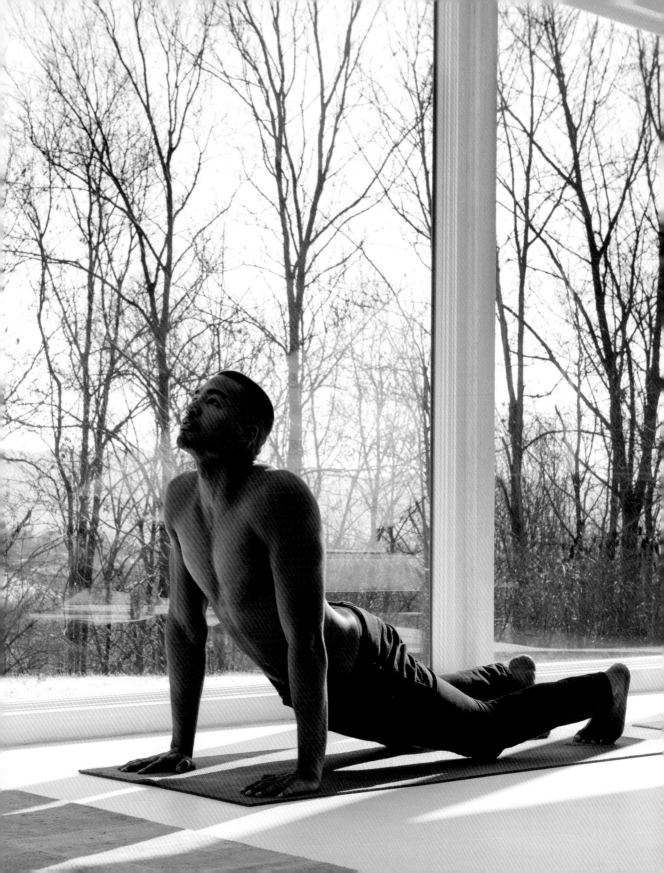

CHAPTER 4

HOW TO START YOUR OWN STRETCHING ROUTINE

In chapter 7, you'll find dozens of ready-made stretching routines perfect for incorporating into your life today. They are specifically designed to take just a few minutes and can be easily modified to fit your activity level and time requirements. You can simply pick one (or more!) based on your needs and dive right in. If you are new to stretching, there are a few things you might want to consider before you get started, like the best place in your home to stretch or how to schedule a stretch sesh into your daily routine. Use these ideas to set yourself up for success:

1 | Find Your Stretching Space

It can be helpful to pick a dedicated spot in your home for stretching since you'll want to have some space. Depending on which body part you are stretching, you're likely going to need more than a yoga mat's worth of space to move around, but having a yoga mat handy is a good place to start. If you are stretching indoors, find a spacious area in your home or room without furniture or clutter. Make sure there are no lamps within arm's length or beautiful vases within kicking distance. Ultimately, you want an environment that makes you feel relaxed and doesn't add any more tension to your body.

If it's easy for you to get up off the ground, the floor is the best starting point since it provides a flat and stable surface from which to begin. For others, getting up and down from the floor may prove challenging, so some stretching can be done standing or even in bed. It really depends on your goals, the muscles you're going to target, and your physical health and mobility.

2 | Put On Something Comfortable

In order to properly stretch, you're going to want to wear clothing that allows you to move and breathe freely. Yoga or elastic pants and tops that are both flexible and breathable are a great place to start. Shorts and short-sleeve (or even better, sleeveless) tops ensure the lowest possibility of clothing getting in the way of your movement. One key: If you are stretching outdoors, make sure you are wearing weather-appropri-

ate clothes. You don't want to feel chilled or cold while stretching, because being cold can cause your muscles to tense up, inhibiting the stretching effect you intend to accomplish.

3 | Set Aside Some Time

It's never fun to feel rushed, and that's especially true when you're stretching. Allow yourself enough time so you can perform your routine in total relaxation. Just how long that routine is depends on a few things, including how many muscles you will be targeting and your specific goals. You will likely need a minimum of 5 to 10 minutes but shouldn't need more than 30.

As for when to stretch, again consider your personal goals and how you feel. While the overall research on stretching shows it is beneficial for health and effective at improving range of motion and joint mobility, especially as we age, it can have negative consequences on athletic performance. Many studies show a reduction in power output of muscles when they have been stretched immediately prior to exercise. And yet studies also show that the improvements in mobility at a joint can be beneficial at injury prevention.

Ultimately, the best time to stretch is anytime you do it. For older individuals who may wake feeling very stiff and achy first thing in the morning, I often recommend starting the day with some gentle stretching to promote blood flow to the muscles and encourage better mobility throughout the day. For younger athletes, it may be helpful to wait until there is already a little blood flow throughout the body and stretch before or after activity, or at the end of the day to wind down. Really, there is no wrong time to stretch unless you are extremely set on achieving your ultimate physical performance. In that case, do dynamic stretching prior to physical activity (rather than static stretching), followed by some static stretching afterward.

4 | Do It Regularly

Stretching, like any practice, should be done regularly if you hope to benefit from its effects long-term. While there are some immediate benefits to stretching, those usually don't last if you don't continue to stretch more regularly. Depending on whether you are stretching because it feels good or because you have an injury that you are rehabilitating, stretching can be done just about every day. If that's too much, try to start with 3 to 5 times a week, and gradually make it more of a daily ritual. Once you see results, you'll know you're doing it right.

5 | Reach a Little Farther (If It Feels Right)

Practice and regular stretching should, by definition, help you progress and become more flexible. There is no exact amount you have to stretch each time you stretch; simply feel your body and allow the progress to reveal itself as you notice increased mobility and reduced tension in your muscles. Generally, stretches can be progressed by taking them a little deeper—sinking into them more, allowing more motion at each joint as that

space becomes available to you. Another way to progress stretching is to do slight variations of stretches. For example, a calf stretch performed by lunging may not be as deep a stretch as if you let your heel hang off the edge of a step.

Also, recognize that muscles don't exist in isolation: They are interconnected chains of tension. In order to maximize the benefits of stretching, make sure you are stretching not just individual muscles but the surrounding musculature as well. This will help promote blood flow throughout the entire body.

ALL ABOUT ACCESSORIES

There are many different accessories out there to help you further the benefits of stretching and improve your comfort and effectiveness as you do it. You can get a perfectly good stretch without any props, but if you would like to try something new, here is a list of just a few of the options out there and how they can best serve you.

Foam Rollers

Foam rollers are light, portable, cylindrical foam tubes or structures that are used often by athletes and physical therapists in the muscle recovery process. While the evidence is mixed on the true effectiveness of foam rolling in helping to heal injuries or improve function, the one area experts seem to agree on is that foam rolling—like stretching—can improve range of motion at a joint.

Foam rollers are relatively cheap and come in different sizes and firmness levels. They work by applying pressure to the muscles and not just physically distorting the tissue slightly, but sending signals to your brain to reduce tension in the body. By rolling over a specific muscle area, this also promotes blood flow to the area. The combination of reducing tension or tone, increasing blood flow, and some stretching that occurs while using a foam roller can help promote gains in range of motion at a stiff joint. Think of it as a self-massage or self-myofascial release.

I usually recommend using a foam roller to anyone aiming to improve their mobility and reduce tension or soreness in a muscle. However, sometimes the positioning needed to effectively use the foam roller can require upper body and core strength and a certain degree of mobility that not everyone has. So, you'll want to check with a physical therapist or health care practitioner if you are physically limited in some way to make sure the foam roller will be an effective tool for you.

Stretching Straps

A stretching strap is another cheap and easy-to-use tool that can help deepen and accommodate certain stretches. A stretching strap is a long strap (usually green) that has multiple loops along it. It can be useful for stretching longer limbs or working on harder-to-reach holds by acting as an extension of your arms. It is similar to a yoga strap, except the addition of the loops allows you to hook the end of your foot or ankle into a strap to prevent sliding while holding a stretch or pose.

I find the stretching strap particularly effective for quad and hamstring stretches, though there are many creative uses of the strap. If you are performing a hamstring stretch lying on your back, the stretching strap allows you to place your foot in one of the loops and hold on to separate sections of the strap by hooking your hands through the loop as you lift your leg up toward the ceiling and hold it there. For people who struggle with tight hamstrings, the strap allows for a more modified or adjustable stretch while allowing your body to stay in a neutral spine position.

Yoga Blocks

If you are doing yoga or performing stretches while seated or standing and reaching toward the ground, yoga blocks can bring the ground up to your hands or hips if your hands and hips can't reach the floor due to stiffness. There are quite a number of ways to use the yoga blocks, depending on what you're trying to achieve. But for anyone who has ever taken a yoga class and felt some of the stretches were a bit too hard to manage, the yoga blocks allow one to self-modify in a group setting when individual attention is not given. Like the foam roller and stretching strap, they are also cheap, small, and simple tools that help get the job done.

Percussive Massage Machines

Some of the newer and most popular tools being used today are the Hypervolt and Theragun, two examples of percussive massage machines. Why? Not only

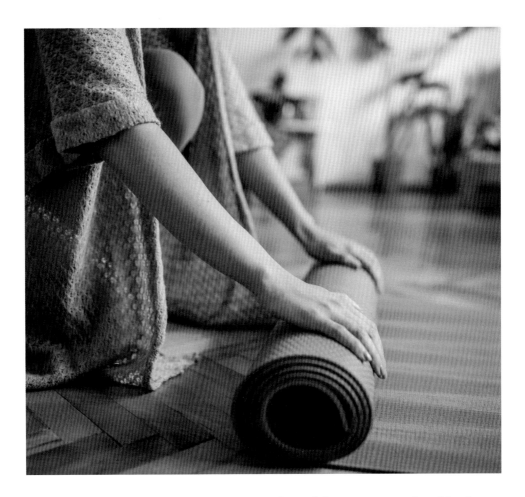

do they feel amazing (think your own handheld masseuse for all those knots and sore spots), but they also seem to be helpful in both activating and stimulating a muscle and promoting blood flow for recovery after a tough workout. And honestly, they just feel fantastic.

While these are the priciest of all the accessories listed, they are a favorite among athletes and nonathletes alike. They are used more often to clear metabolic waste products that pool in the body after a tough workout, but by mechanically stimulating the soft tissue through battery-operated rapid pulse pressure, they are like a turbo-charged foam roller, promoting blood flow and stimulating receptors in the body to help reduce soreness and tension while allowing for gains in mobility.

When it comes to creating your own stretching routine, let this be your guiding light: Listen to your body. You will start to notice in the minutes, hours, and days after stretching how it affects your body. Pay attention to these signals and gently adjust as needed.

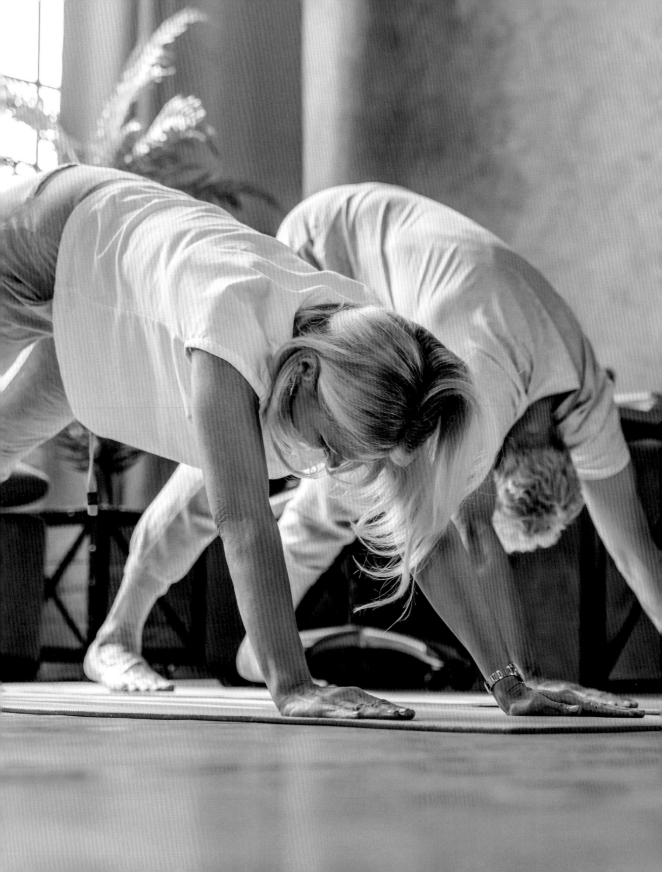

CHAPTER 5

ADJUSTING YOUR STRETCHING ROUTINE

Unlike some physical activities, stretching is something you can stick with for life. For the most part, you can't get sidelined by an injury or lose your momentum. In fact, if you get injured, stretching may be one of the first things your doctor recommends!

Over time, you may find that you want to adjust your stretching routine. You might cycle through dozens of different stretches before you find those that truly put a spring in your step (you'll know when you find them!). Maybe it is some neck rolls, calf stretches, and downward dogs that work the kinks out of your body. Ultimately, you're going to want to focus on the areas that need individual attention in your unique body. Everyone is different, and everyone's points of restriction or pain can be different too. Whether you have a history of certain injuries or body positioning or a new area of concern, you're going to want to know and understand your own body to determine where to focus your attention.

That said, over time, things usually change. If you are effectively performing your stretches, you will likely not need to stretch the same muscle every time. There is so much variety in life and in our movement patterns that it is possible you will need to vary your stretching routine as time goes on. It could even happen from season to season. For example, you may shovel snow in the winter but go all of spring without ever repeating that same motion pattern. When that happens, again, pay close attention to the muscles at work, and pivot your stretching sessions to include these newly active muscles.

Other changes might require a closer lens. Here's how to tailor your routine for whatever life brings your way.

As You Age

You've no doubt noticed that your body changes as you get older. The effects of aging—and how fast they come on—depend on lifestyle and genetics, among other things. There are differences that will be more specific to each person based on the way they have been moving, eating, and living for decades. These unique factors should be considered as you evolve your stretching habits over the years.

Of course, there are some general assumptions that can be made about an 80-year-old's body and a 15-year-old's body. Certain natural, degenerative processes occur in the body with age and can affect the way we move and stretch. One of the most well-known of these is osteoarthritis (OA). OA is a degenera-

tion of the smooth cartilaginous surface at the end of a bone. Some people might experience OA in their 50s, while others might not feel its effects until their 70s. But, for the most part, some OA is likely to occur in just about everyone over time.

OA can cause inflammation and pain as well as physical changes to the joint that change the way we move. It can impact any joint in the body from your neck to your hips to your back. This type of pain usually arises during everyday movements such as going up and down stairs, getting up from a low chair, turning your head to the side to cross the street, or employing fine-motor skills with your hands such as using scissors. While OA can be felt at rest, it is usually felt most after activity and at the end range of certain movements, such as bending the knees past a certain point or trying to grip and carry a small, heavy object. To some degree, it is a part of the natural aging process, but the extent to which it develops is more affected by lifestyle.

As you age, you should keep up healthy movement patterns and practices to maintain mobility in your joints. Pay particular attention to the shoulder and hip joints, which are two of the joints that—when healthy and young—have the most mobility in the body. While some joints, like the knee joint, are predominantly a hinge joint that just bends and straightens, the shoulder and hip joints are ball-and-socket joints that allow movement up, down, forward, backward, to the side, and all around.

This mobility can be greatly impacted by pain or weakness over time. To some extent the old saying is true: If you don't use it, you lose it (mobility, that is).

As mentioned before, everything is connected. You can't expect perfect shoulder mobility as you age if your upper back begins to round and your head juts forward. These changes to body alignment can contribute to deficits in mobility and strength, and with them function. So, a full-body stretching routine and an active, mobile lifestyle that addresses the whole you—not just one body part at a time—is usually the best bet for maintaining mobility as you age. Diet, general health, and sleep quality along with many other variables play a significant role as well. But with so many ways to move, maintain strength, and maintain flexibility, there is bound to be one that feels right for you and your body. And that's the one you should be doing. Ultimately, if we don't enjoy moving and exercising, we won't do it, so try different options until you find what's right for you. Movement is a privilege; it should not feel like a chore.

When Injuries Arise

Most—but not all—injuries develop over time. They are the result of patterns of movement and not sudden trauma. These types of injuries, commonly known as overuse injuries or tendinopathies, are the most treatable and avoidable injuries. Acute injuries, such as stepping in a pothole and twisting an ankle, are harder to predict or avoid, unfortunately. But thankfully, they can still heal with the proper treatment and guidance.

Get ahead of overuse injuries by being mindful of the sensations you experience in your body on a daily basis. Take note of how your joints feel, how certain movements such as squatting, standing, walking, reaching for the upper shelf, carrying heavy things, or bending down to get up and down from the floor feel. Getting to know your baseline can make it easier to notice when your body is whispering that something is not right. Is something difficult to do that wasn't before? Does it feel stiff? Is it extra labor intensive suddenly? If the answer is yes, see if you can add new stretches or strengthening exercises to your routine before this whisper becomes a loud scream. It is much easier to address issues when they are minor tightness or stiffness than when they become more acute. Patterns of movement can form, and when you feel something is "off," that's a good signal that you might need to break up the pattern or it will turn into a full-blown injury. Noticing the warning signs before an injury occurs can help you manage many aches and pains and hopefully prevent worsening symptoms.

If you suspect an injury or are experiencing pain, see a physical therapist or orthopedist early on. Don't wait too long, as some injuries such as knee pain or hip pain can lead to a spiral of problems if not addressed early. Imagine pain in one knee causes you to avoid putting weight on it, so you start to limp

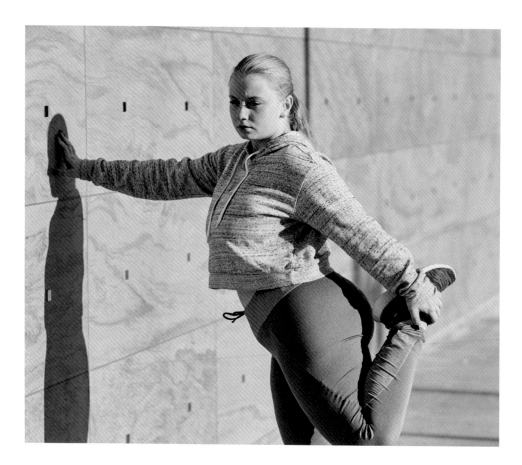

a little. This leads to strained walking, which causes weakness in that side (since you're avoiding using it) and pain in your opposite-side lower back or hip from walking funny.

In other words, one small ache or pain can lead to a cascade of issues if not addressed. So, get to a specialist early on, and they will guide you toward the right exercise routine to help you improve your mobility and strength and likely protect you from future injury by doing a complete assessment of your movement, strength, and function.

For Your Everyday Life

It might seem like adding a stretching routine to your already packed to-do list is just wishful thinking. But there are many ways you can incorporate smart movement into your daily life. I like to find ways to stretch on the go or when fully dressed, often sneaking in a stretch while doing things I already do in my day. For example, while waiting for the subway or a light to change, put one foot in front of the other for a quick lunge to stretch the calves. Next time you're standing in line at a store, grab your hands behind your back and open up the chest muscles. And when you've been sitting in your chair for hours, try leaning your upper back over the top of the chair and letting your ribs and belly open up. Cross one leg over the other and lean forward to stretch your hip. Though small, these habits can have a positive impact on our mobility.

For more stretches you can sneak into your daily routine, check out the list below:

STANDING:
- Calf Stretches (p. 105)
- Pec Stretches (p. 92)
- Neck Stretches (p. 114)
- Wrist Stretches (p. 77)

SITTING:
- Sitting Thoracic Extension Stretch (p. 91)
- Sitting Figure Four Stretch (p. 96)
- Knee to Chest Stretch (p. 95)
- Sitting Hamstring Stretch (p. 108)
- Overhead Reach with Mini Side Bend (p. 87)

WALKING:
- Arm Swings (p. 120)
- Butt Kicks (p. 122)
- Leg Swings (p. 127)
- High Knees (p. 125)

If you don't have time for a full-blown stretch session, consider which of these three positions (sitting, standing, and walking) you spend the most time in, and start with that list of stretches before making time for others. Even just 5 minutes can make a difference. If you can't squeeze in a couple of minutes, it is okay to skip a day or two of stretching. You can still make progress (some is better than none). However, research does indicate that regular stretching is needed for optimal gains in mobility, so try not to go weeks without it.

WHY QUICK STRETCHES COUNT

According to the American College of Sports Medicine (ACSM), adults should stretch 2-3 days per week, addressing all the major muscle groups in their body, in order to achieve gains in range of motion. That might sound like a lot, but you only need to hold each stretch for 10-30 seconds at a time for 2-4 reps until you've reached at least 60 seconds of total stretching time for a particular joint. Studies have shown that there is no increase in muscle elongation after 2-4 reps, so a short stretch session is really all you need!

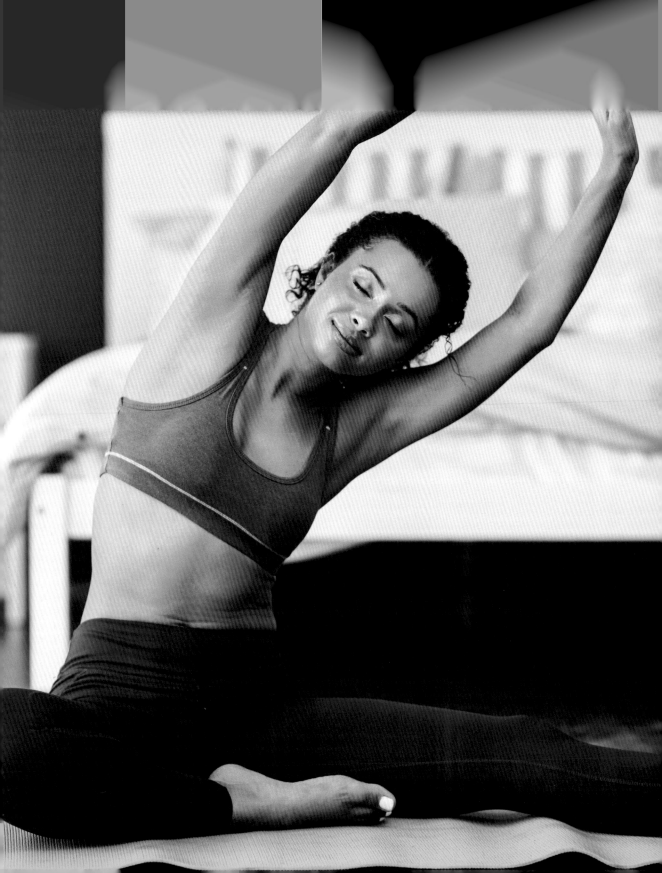

CHAPTER 6

HOW TO STAY LIMBER & PAIN-FREE FOR LIFE

Ultimately, the best remedy for aches and pains is a solid, proactive plan for avoiding them in the first place. Some parts of aging are unavoidable, but there are actions you can take to delay their arrival and minimize their impact. Gradually adding these little healthy habits to your daily routine can help you prevent pain and stiffness so you can move through life with ease.

Stand More

You know that sitting too long too frequently can negatively impact your health, from limiting your mobility to increasing your risk for heart problems and blood clots. It's even been linked to your mood, with studies showing a connection between depression risk and time spent being sedentary. But making time to stand more can be difficult if your job has you tethered to a desk. If a standing work station isn't in the cards for you, make it a goal to get up from your chair more often. You can also set a timer on your phone for every 30 minutes so you don't forget to stand up, get the blood flowing, and move between bouts of productivity. It may even help you get things done.

Practice Good Posture

If you are glued to a chair all day, you can still mitigate some of its negative impacts by sitting up straight. Sitting in general can put up to 40% more pressure on your back than standing. Slouching on top of that can trigger back and neck pain and decrease your mobility. Not sure what perfect posture feels like? Imagine a string pulling you straight up from your spine, and allow your shoulders to roll back slightly.

Try a New Sleeping Position

Despite all the advances in mattresses, pillows, and sleep tech, there is still a good chance that you will leave your bed feeling stiff and tight in the morning. After all, you are spending about 8 hours in the exact same position (or some variation of lying down). The position that will best support your needs is very personal. For example, if you have lower back pain, try sleeping on your side with a pillow between your legs. This will help keep your back straight in relation to your hips and pelvis. The one position to avoid? In most cases, that's sleeping on your stomach. It forces your head to twist either to the left or right, potentially causing neck strain.

Sneak in a Variety of Movement

Remember how moving your body in a limited range of motion can lead to mobility issues over time? Dedicating time to stretching is a great way to make sure your muscles get the movement they need, but you can also fully realize your mobility in little ways throughout your day. Simple actions, like taking the stairs, walking while talking on the phone, or parking farther away from the grocery store, all get your body moving and help maintain good mobility.

Eat for Joint Health

The right diet can actually give your bones a boost and help ease creaky joints that can come with aging. Maintaining a healthy weight is one of the best things you can do for your joints, but integrating special joint-healthy foods into your diet can also be beneficial. Foods high in calcium, collagen, omega-3s, magnesium, or vitamins D, C, or K may be able to help support bone and joint health. As for what to start stocking in your kitchen, here are some versatile staples:

Turmeric

Turmeric is great for combating inflammation thanks to a special compound known as curcumin. Studies have linked curcumin to arthritis relief and the potential for improved joint health. Try sprinkling some on scrambled eggs or your favorite roasted vegetable dish for a little inflammation-fighting power.

Fortified Milk

Milk fortified with vitamin D is a great way to get a dose of joint-friendly nutrients. Vitamin D is crucial to helping your body absorb calcium, which is also essential to building strong bones and joints.

Blueberries

The polyphenols in blueberries may help relieve joint pain from arthritis, according to studies. Plus, one serving of this sweet berry packs 16% of your daily recommended vitamin C, which helps promote the production of collagen.

Bell Peppers

These colorful peppers are actually packed with vitamin C—one medium pepper contains more than a day's worth of the nutrient.

Mushrooms

One of the few whole food sources of vitamin D, mushrooms are a great way to support joint health. Because vitamin D works hand-in-hand with calcium, try pairing some mushrooms with calcium-rich cheese for a bone-healthy combo.

Minimize Stress

Finally, identify avoidable stressors in your life. Stress creates tension in the body. It's almost like your body's way of preparing you for impact. Yes, stretching helps relieve it, but if you can sidestep stressors from the start, you can help make sure you never end the day with your shoulders tensed up to your ears. Try to take note of what causes stress in your life so you notice patterns. Even if you can't eliminate the culprits, you will still be better prepared to handle them mindfully (and hopefully with a little less fist clenching!).

NEED-TO-KNOW NUTRIENTS

Happy joints start in the kitchen. Here's exactly how a well-rounded diet can help keep your body moving pain-free.

CALCIUM

Used by your body to build strong bones; not found naturally in the body

VITAMIN D

Aids in the absorption of calcium

COLLAGEN

Also used to build strong bones; may help maintain joint health

VITAMIN C

Promotes collagen synthesis

OMEGA-3S

Healthy fatty acid that can help fight inflammation

MAGNESIUM

Contributes to bone density

VITAMIN K

Helps transport calcium to bones

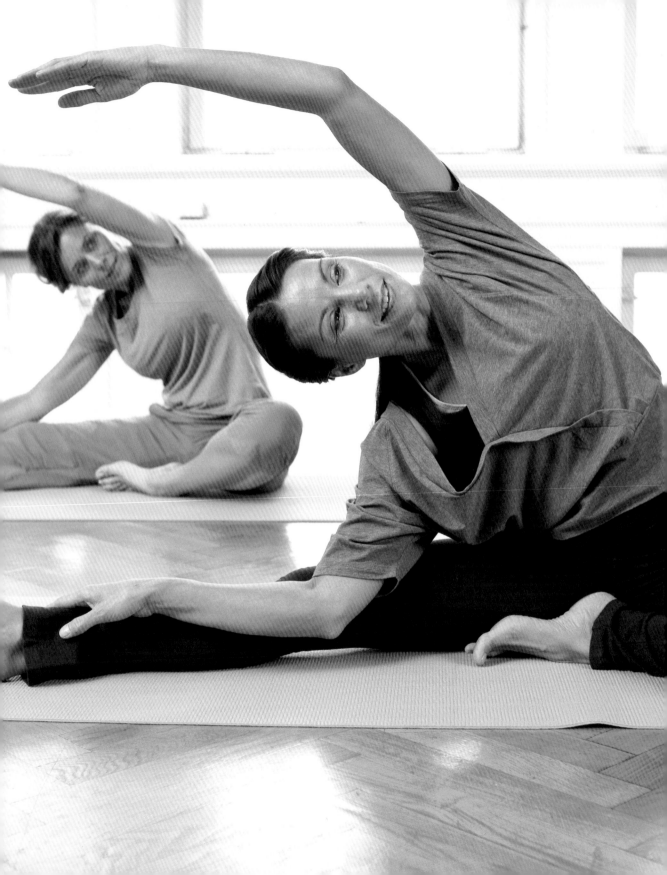

CHAPTER 7

STRETCHING
ROUTINES

The best stretching routine is the one you will actually want to do day in and day out. The options here are designed to be just that. They are short and simple yet incredibly effective. Just a couple minutes of these exercises will leave you feeling ready to move in whatever way life requires.

In most cases, you will only need to master three or four stretches because the moves shown here are multitaskers. For example, the same stretch that can help relieve your back pain can also help you unwind into total relaxation before bed. (Hint: It's cat-camel.) And the hamstring stretch on page 108 can not only prime your body for a walk but also soothe creaky knees and improve your flexibility. Test different routines until you find the one (or ones!) that makes you feel your best. And don't worry if you haven't stretched a muscle since high school gym class. These routines are suitable for both total beginners and seasoned "stretchers." Though if you want to ease your way into this new way of moving, the beginner's series on the next page is the perfect place to start!

The key for beginners: Take things slowly. Start by really learning to get in touch with your body and the signals it's giving you. When you lean into your first stretch, whether it's a neck stretch or a hip stretch, pay attention to what feels good, what feels mildly uncomfortable, and what you'd consider to be painful. No stretch should feel painful. Take extra time during each position for breathwork, relaxation, and self-assessment. Some body parts might feel extremely stiff and tight while others pose no problem.

As you observe these sensations in each body part, you will determine your limits of mobility. Appreciate them, and don't force yourself past them. The stretches listed here are great for exploring your range of motion and identifying your body's comfort zone, which will help guide you through any routine in this book.

A. Cat-Camel (p. 79)
B. Any Hamstring Stretch (p. 108)
C. Calf Stretch (p. 105)
D. Downward Dog (p. 107)
E. Standing Pec Stretch (p. 92)

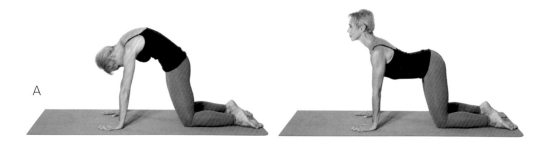

A

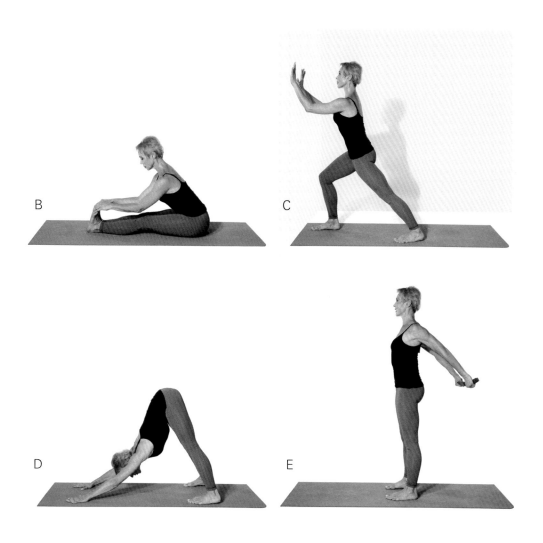

B

C

D

E

Improving flexibility is one of the main purposes of stretching. Think of it as practice, not a one-off routine. Becoming more flexible doesn't happen in one session—it takes time. You'll need to stretch the same joints at least 3 times per week to make lasting progress. Progressing your flexibility also requires holding each stretch up to 30 seconds and repeating it 2 to 4 times. For improved general flexibility, start with the larger muscle groups such as the hips, shoulders, and spine. Then home in on the smaller, more specific muscles where restrictions are felt.

Follow this routine regularly, holding each position for up to 30 seconds and repeating 2 to 4 times, for greater flexibility top to bottom.

A. Any Hamstring Stretch (p. 108)
B. Butterfly Stretch (p. 94)
C. Figure Four Stretch (p. 96)
D. Side-Lying Thoracic Rotation (p. 89)
E. Double Knee to Chest Stretch (p. 97)
F. Lunge Stretch with Overhead Reach (p. 101)
G. Lying-Down Pec Stretch (p. 92)

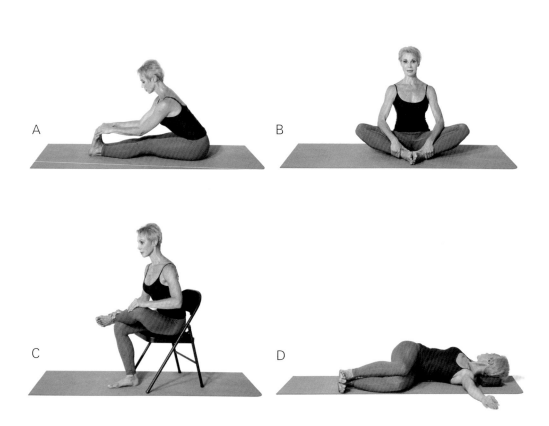

A

B

C

D

E 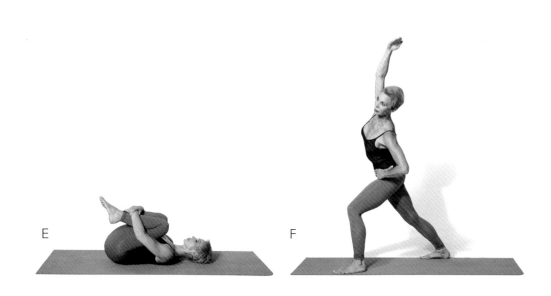 F

G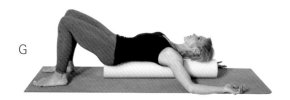

TO REACH A GOAL / ENERGY

Dynamic stretches, which are stretches performed while in motion, are great for promoting blood flow and, with that, increasing energy levels. Although static stretching can boost circulation if you transition between poses without rest (like in a yoga flow), dynamic stretching gets your blood pumping in two ways: both during the transition between stretches and in the stretch itself. Studies have even shown that it can improve power and running performance. How is that for an energy boost? Try this stretching routine in the sequence listed next time you need a pick-me-up.

A. Downward Dog to Cobra (p. 123)
B. High Knees (p. 125)
C. Walking Lunges (p. 132)
D. Arm Swings (p. 120)

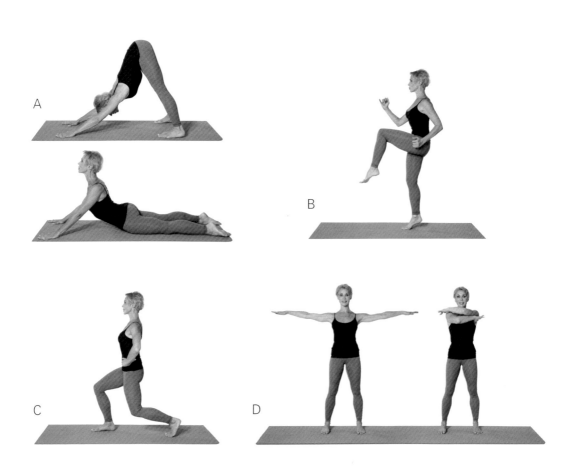

The best stretches to improve posture depend on what particular positions your body is collapsing into when you're tired. The most common culprits of poor posture include weakness—not just tightness—of certain muscles, though tightness in one place can contribute to weakness in another. For example, tightness in the chest can encourage the shoulders to round forward, leading to a simultaneous weakness in the muscles between the shoulder blades, which are meant to hold the shoulders upright and back. While strengthening is an important part of improving posture, stretching is also crucial to helping you stand tall. Be sure to work these moves into your routine:

A. Any Pec Stretch (p. 92)
B. Lunge or Hip Stretch Off Elevated Surface (p. 100, 102)
C. Sitting Thoracic Extension Stretch (p. 91)

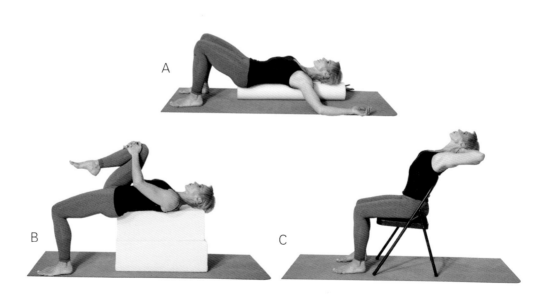

Simply pausing to perform static stretches can be great for promoting relaxation. Stretches that are held in comforting positions, such as child's pose and double knee to chest stretch, can help promote relaxation and direct your focus on breathwork while you allow the muscles to gently elongate. All stretching can be relaxing to some extent, but static stretching is ideal for bringing awareness to your body and your breathing, becoming almost meditative in the process. Give these stretches a go whenever work or life gets stressful.

A. Double Knee to Chest Stretch (p. 97)
B. Child's Pose (p. 81)
C. Lower Trunk Rotation (p. 84)
D. Lying-Down Pec Stretch (p. 92)
E. Cat-Camel (p. 79)

A

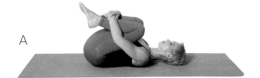

B

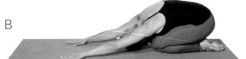

C

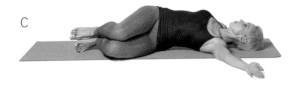

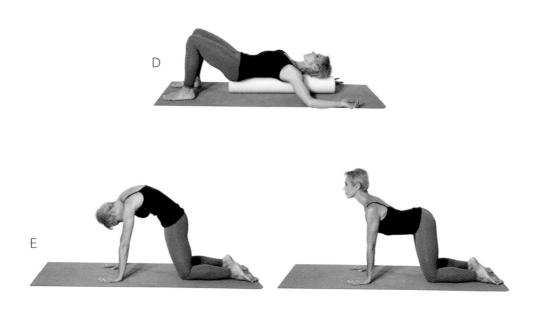

D

E

AS YOU AGE / 40+

Everyone's body ages at a slightly different rate, but one thing is for sure: Once you're over 40, you are likely to see some changes in your mobility as compared to when you were in your 20s. You might start to notice aches and pains in your lower back, neck, shoulders, hips, and knees, or the onset of arthritis. After 40+ years of being an active human, there is likely to be some wear and tear on the surface of the joints. But it doesn't have to slow you down if you counter it with a smart stretching routine. The key for those over 40 is to maintain mobility and flexibility and not let stiffness take over. Focus on stretching the large muscles that cross the hips (quads, iliopsoas, glutes, and hamstrings) as well as the muscles of the chest and shoulder girdle (pecs, traps, and biceps). A good basic routine for those over 40 can include:

A. Any Hamstring Stretch (p. 108)
B. Any Figure Four Stretch (p. 96)
C. Hip Stretch Off Elevated Surface (p. 102)
D. Any Pec Stretch (p. 92)

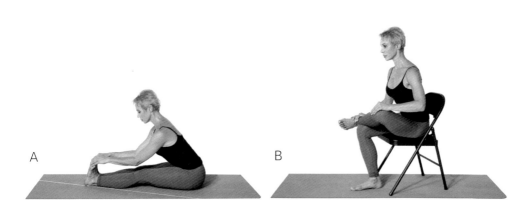

A

B

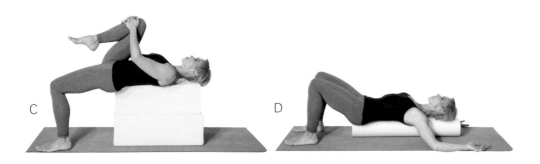

C

D

People over 65 often develop age-related conditions that can be helped by stretching. For example, as we age, the spine tends to prefer a more flexed or curled forward position versus extension (think fetal position over cobra pose). This is due to narrowing of the spinal canal and shrinking disc space between each vertebra. Flexing forward helps open up the spinal canal, relieving pressure on the nerves, which are often a culprit of pain. Generally speaking, if you're over 65, you'll want to focus on more flexion-based positions, which require your back to fold forward, like when you hug your knees to your chest (the opposite is when you extend your spine, as back bends or any version of a cobra pose require). There are exceptions to every rule, but this is a good general one to go by. Here is a good flexion-based stretching routine:

A. Double Knee to Chest Stretch (p. 97)
B. Lower Trunk Rotation (p. 84)
C. Any Hamstring Stretch (p. 108)
D. Side-Lying Thoracic Rotation (p. 89)

A

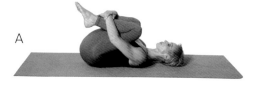

B

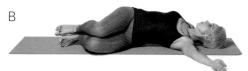

C

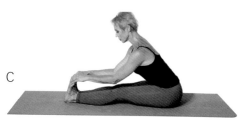

D

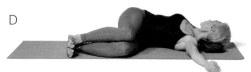

> *Be sure to talk to your doctor about any pain you are experiencing before using the stretches in this section.*

As mentioned in chapter 3, back pain often has to do with more than just your back. Tension in the glutes and hamstrings as well as the pecs and muscles of the anterior hip can cause discomfort throughout your back by affecting your overall alignment, body mechanics, and strength. Depending on the individual and type of tension, back pain can make it difficult to stand, so here are some stretches that can be done in more relaxed positions.

A. Lying-Down Hamstring Stretch (p. 108)
B. Standing Hamstring Stretch (p. 108)
C. Quad Stretch (p. 113)
D. Hip Stretch Off Elevated Surface (p. 102)
E. Cat-Camel (p. 79)

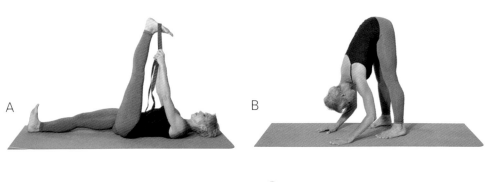

A

B

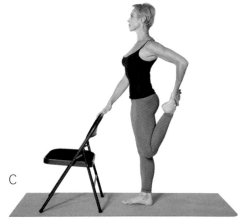

C

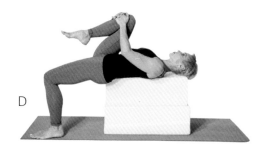

D

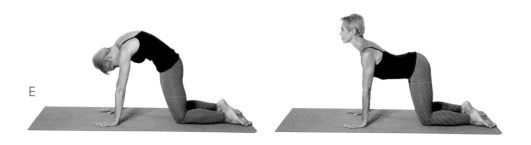

E

Everything from your workout to your weight can impact hip pain, so it's important to have a stretching routine to combat it. These stretches provide a multifaceted approach so you aren't just stretching one area and neglecting the rest.

A. Any Hamstring Stretch (p. 108)
B. Any Figure Four Stretch (p. 96)
C. Hip Stretch Off Elevated Surface (p. 102)
D. Butterfly Stretch (p. 94)
E. Double Knee to Chest Stretch (p. 97)
F. Cross-Body Knee to Chest Stretch (p. 83)
G. Lunge Stretch with Overhead Reach (p. 101)

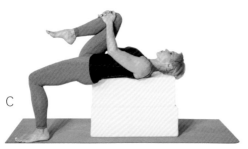

A

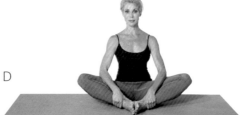

B

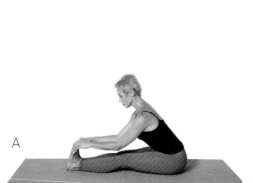

C

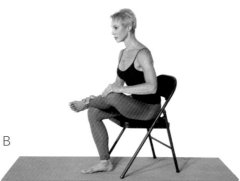

D

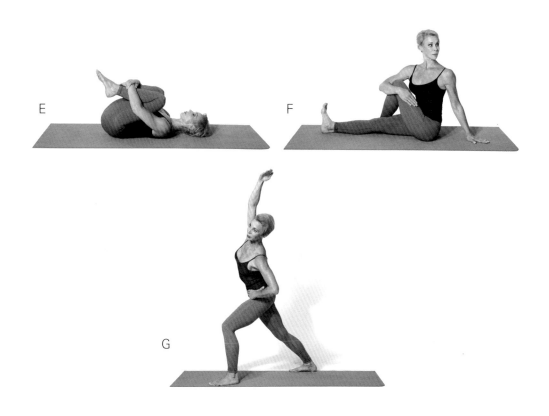

TO EASE SPECIFIC PAINS / KNEE PAIN

Remember, stretching the muscles around your knee, such as the hamstring, gastrocnemius, and quadriceps, is a good place to start addressing pain in this area. This quick and easy routine will help unwind tightness and ease aches.

A. Any Hamstring Stretch (p. 108)
B. Quad Stretch (p. 113)
C. IT Band "Stretch" (p. 99)
D. Calf Stretch (p. 105)

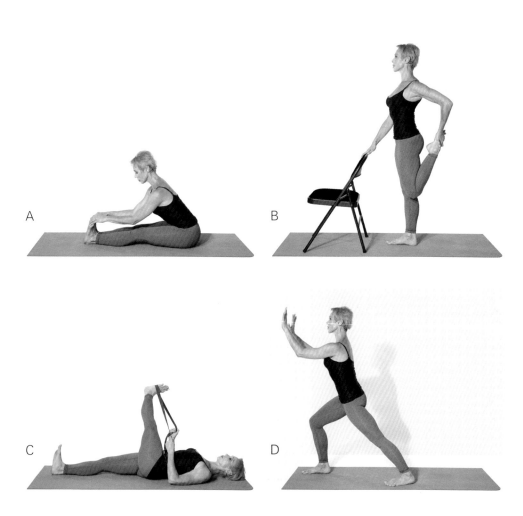

A

B

C

D

Whether you're hunching over a computer all day or staring down at your phone, you likely experience neck pain from time to time. These simple stretches are quick enough to do throughout your day to break up hours of screen time and nix neck pain before it gets worse.

A. Upper Trap Stretch (p. 117)
B. Chin Tucks (p. 114)
C. Any Pec Stretch (p. 92)
D. Sitting Thoracic Extension Stretch (p. 91)

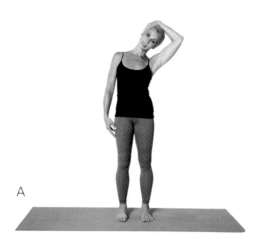

A

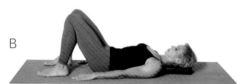

B

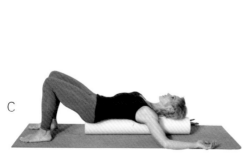

C

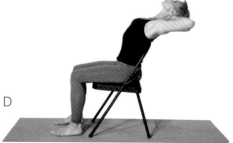

D

Sciatica is leg pain caused by a pinched nerve in the lower back. Although the pangs begin in nerve roots located on either side of the lower spine, they then course through the sciatic nerve, which runs the length of each leg from the buttock down to the foot. Check with a medical professional before starting any plan, and then check out these stretches to help alleviate pain.

A. Any Hamstring Stretch (p. 108)
B. Hip Stretch Off Elevated Surface (p. 102)
C. Any Figure Four Stretch (p. 96)
D. Double Knee to Chest Stretch (p. 97)
E. Prone Press-Up Stretch (p. 88)

A

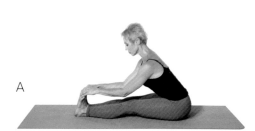

B

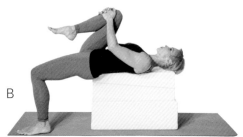

C

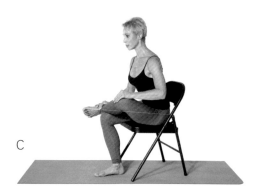

D

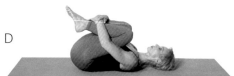

E

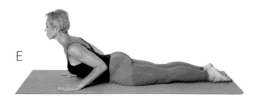

Your chest muscles, neck, arms, and upper back are all connected to your shoulders, so focusing on these areas will help undo a day that has left your shoulders tensed up to your ears. Try these moves next time that kind of day rolls around:

A. Any Pec Stretch (p. 92)
B. Arm Across Chest Stretch (p. 119)
C. Biceps Stretch (p. 76)
D. Sitting Thoracic Extension Stretch (p. 91)

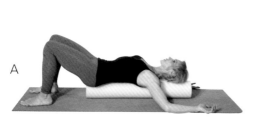

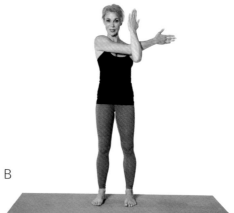

A

B

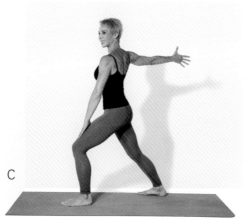

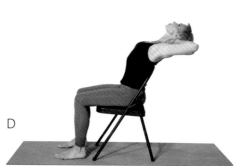

C

D

Stretching can help improve mobility, which becomes more and more limited by stiff and creaky joints affected by arthritis. If you go too long without a proper stretching routine, you are likely to develop increased pain and reduced function. Osteoarthritis tends to affect the joints of the hips, knees, lower back, and shoulders, so focus on stretching these areas regularly. Also, continue to move! Movement promotes blood flow and joint lubrication, both of which can be beneficial to those with arthritis.

When we stop moving, the stiffness and joint restrictions increase, and this makes it harder to get back to moving when we are ready. So, a continuous, regular exercise routine that includes ample static stretching, like this routine, is always a good idea.

A. Any Hamstring Stretch (p. 108)
B. Double Knee to Chest Stretch (p. 97)
C. Any Figure Four Stretch (p. 96)
D. Calf Stretch (p. 105)
E. Side-Lying Thoracic Rotation (p. 89)

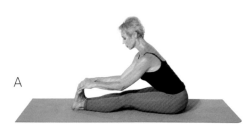

A

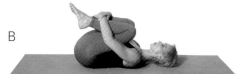

B

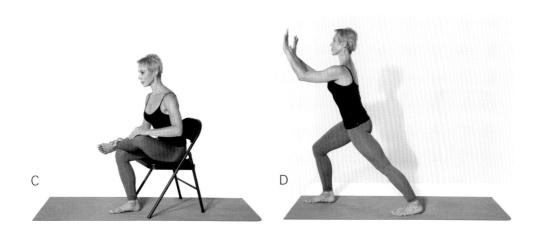

C

D

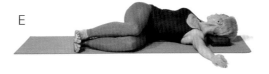

E

BEFORE AND AFTER WORKING OUT

Warming up before a workout quite literally means warming up the muscles and promoting blood flow. In most cases, you'll want to use dynamic stretches to prep your body for exercise. Research has shown that static stretching may negatively impact your muscles' power output. So, unless your workout requires significant joint flexibility (like gymnastics or dance), stick with dynamic. Exactly which dynamic moves you need depends on the activity you're preparing for. If you're going swimming, focus on arm and upper body stretches (like the kind you've probably seen Olympic swimmers perform before a competition). If you're going for a run, concentrate on quick jumping movements or kicking motions targeting the legs. If you're going for a power walk, warming up could entail some simple calf stretches before hitting the pavement. Bottom line: The muscles you plan to use are the ones you're going to want to warm up.

Stretching is also important after a workout. It can help your body cool down and bring your heart rate back to where it was pre-exercise. Therefore, dynamic stretches, which increase blood flow and heart rate, aren't the best choice. Static stretches, which involve slowly easing into a position, allow your muscles to relax, your breathing to slow, and your body to return to its natural state. If you're a runner, this could mean doing a calf stretch on the edge of a step or lying on your back with your feet up against a wall. By slowing down your activity level and your breathing, you can reduce your heart rate after an activity and, in turn, reduce the heat caused by increased blood flow to your muscles. For specific stretching routines based on activity, check out the next few pages.

According to research, static stretching prior to running may reduce athletic performance and does not necessarily prevent injury. However, a little dynamic stretching has proven to be beneficial for improving range of motion without reducing athletic performance and power. So, if you plan to run, start with a dynamic warmup before heading out. If anything is tight after you finish your route, you can do some static stretching to cool down and reduce tension in the muscles.

DYNAMIC STRETCHES FOR RUNNERS
Repeat each one for 30 to 60 seconds or as many reps as indicated.
   A. Leg Swings (p. 127)
   B. Walking Lunges (p. 132)
   C. High Knees (p. 125)
   D. Butt Kicks (p. 122)

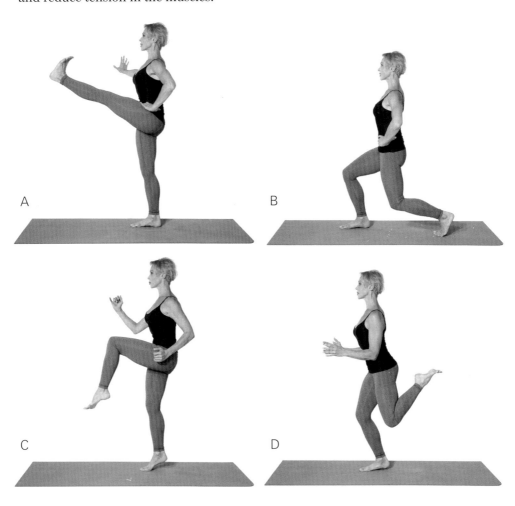

A

B

C

D

STATIC STRETCHES FOR RUNNERS

A. Any Hamstring Stretch (p. 108)
B. Quad Stretch (p. 113)
C. Calf Stretch (p. 105)
D. Lunge Stretch with Overhead Reach (p. 101)
E. Any Figure Four Stretch (p. 96)
F. Any Pec Stretch (p. 92)

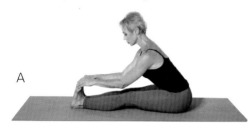

A

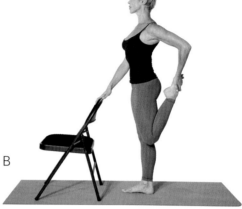

B

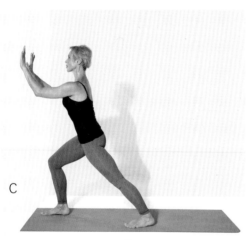

C

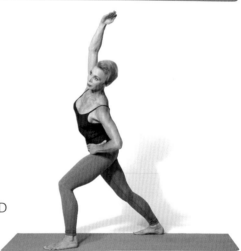

D

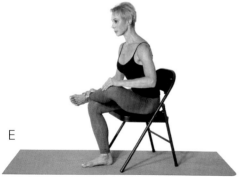

E

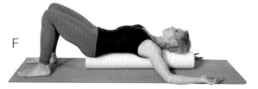

F

Walking is one of the best exercises out there. It has been shown to improve mood, promote weight loss, and even help reduce the risk of chronic disease. Before heading out for a walk, you'll want to perform a few static stretches to limber up the muscles you'll be using, which are primarily your legs. As previously mentioned, dynamic stretches are typically the preferred warmup method for most athletic activities because they do not impact your muscles' power output. However, because walking doesn't require a lot of muscle power (especially compared to, say, performing sprints), static stretching is the way to go. Plus, static stretches are gentler on your body, which may be helpful for those who walk as an alternative to more intensive exercise.

A. Any Hamstring Stretch (p. 108)
B. Calf Stretch (p. 105)
C. Lunge Stretch with Overhead Reach (p. 101)

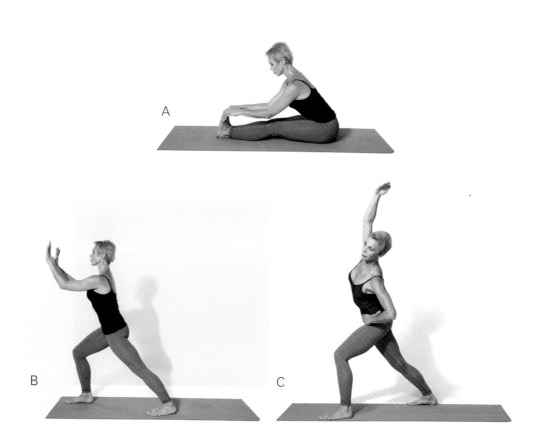

Swimmers use their bodies in ways that differ from runners and walkers. You'll need your arms and legs to be loose for relaxed and comfortable strokes. Swimming itself can be a great warmup for the muscles, but it's important to perform a few stretches before you jump in the water. Try these exercises to get the blood flowing and the body ready for some laps.

A. Arm Swings (p. 120)
B. Trunk Twists (p. 133)
C. Leg Swings (p. 127)

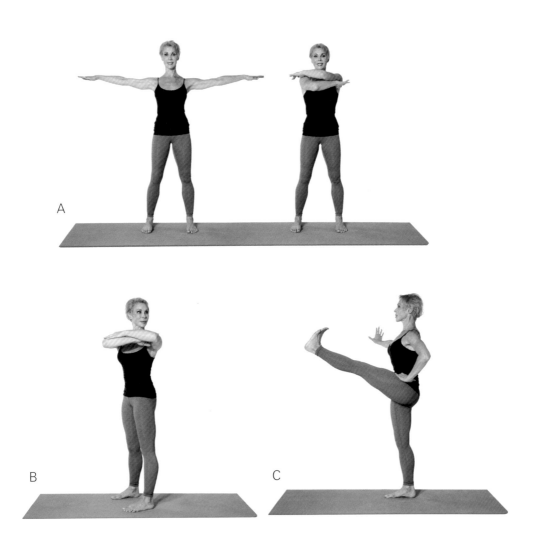

Hiking on uneven terrain requires many of the same muscles as walking but to a more intense degree. For example, if you're trekking up a winding mountain trail, your calves will be working harder than they would on a flat sidewalk. Steep ups and downs can require more mobility in your hips, knees, and ankles, and your muscles are likely going to be more prone to fatigue due to the higher demand on them. Focus on stretches that mimic the way your body will need to move on the trail, like these:

A. Marching in Place (p. 128)
B. Calf Stretch (p. 105)
C. Lunge Stretch with Overhead Reach (p. 101)
D. Walking Lunges (p. 132)

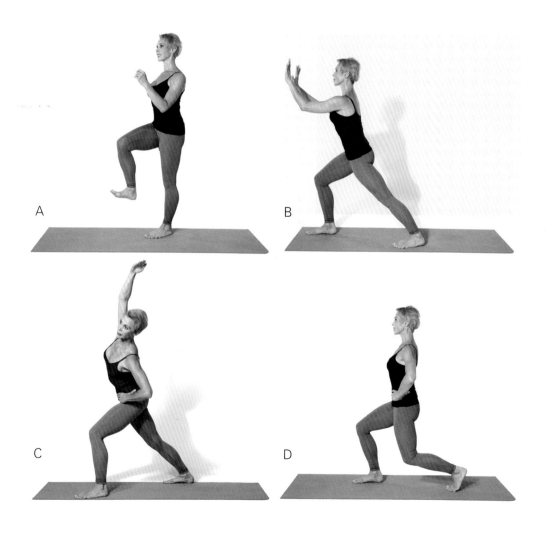

Spending hours on end in a chair is one of the most common causes of stiffness, aches, and pains in the body. When you look at your body in a sitting position, you can likely guess which muscles might begin to tighten. Sitting requires you to fold your hips to about a 90-degree angle. If you're in that position for hours, you'll probably notice tension in your hips. You might find that your shoulders tend to round forward, and your head juts out to get closer to your screen. It is also likely that your arms will be out in front of you to access your keyboard, which further reinforces this forward, rounded shoulder position. It's a recipe for tense muscles. Luckily, there are plenty of stretches you can do to help counter these closed, folded positions—and some don't even require you to get up! Try these exercises the next time you're feeling the effects of sitting all day:

A. Any Pec Stretch (p. 92)
B. Sitting Thoracic Extension Stretch (p. 91)
C. Wrist Stretch (p. 77)
D. Sitting Figure Four Stretch (p. 96)
E. Lunge Stretch with Overhead Reach (p. 101)

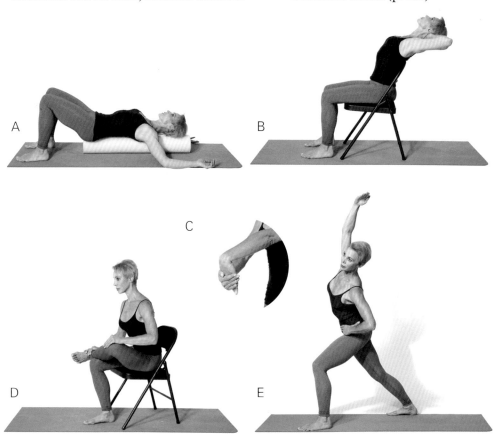

Standing for prolonged periods of time can lead to tight and tired legs. While resting your legs and kicking your feet up is one of the best ways to give your legs a break, stretching can also be helpful, as some muscles can tighten up when fatigued. Most people, depending on what kind of footwear they've been walking around in, will feel tightness particularly in the calves and potentially in the bottom of their feet. Try these stretches to ease the aches.

A. Calf Stretch (p. 105)
B. Plantar Fascia Rollout (p. 110)

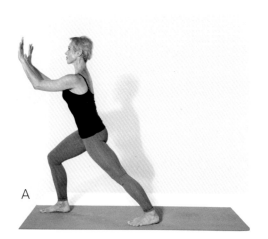

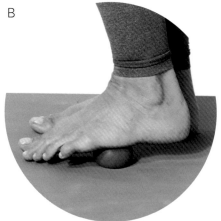

USING ACCESSORIES

Accessories provide a great way to adjust the intensity of a stretch beyond what your body is capable of on its own. Once you start using tools, like foam rollers or stretching straps, you may find one works best for your unique needs. Here are a couple easy ways to get started with these tools and incorporate them into a routine:

FOAM ROLLER STRETCHES

A. Lying-Down Thoracic Extension Stretch (p. 91)
B. Lying-Down Pec Stretch (p. 92)
C. Neck Extension over Foam Roller (p. 115)

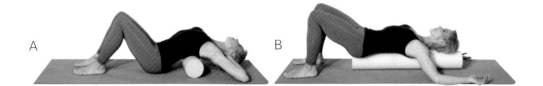

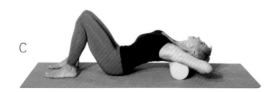

STRAP STRETCHES

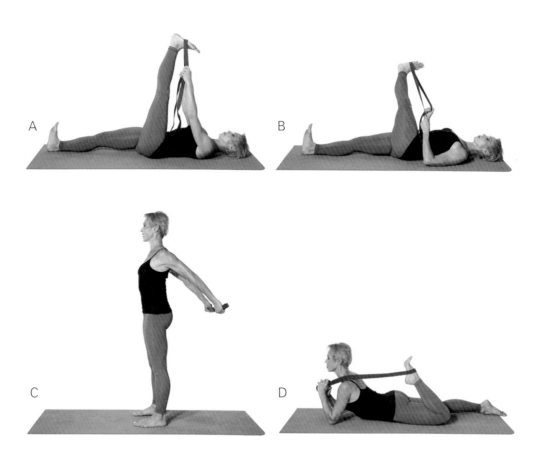

A

B

C

D

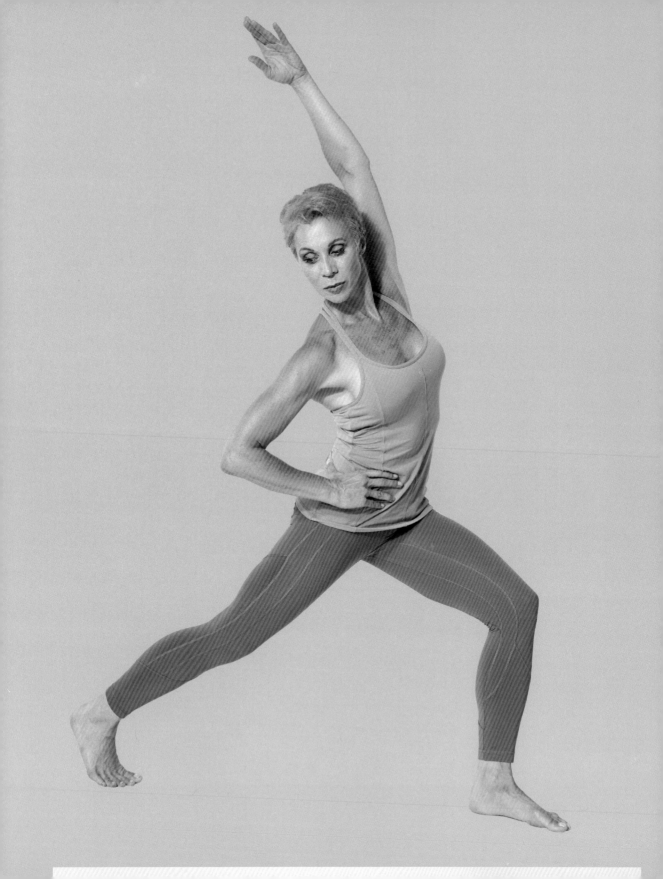

CHAPTER 8

STRETCHING
GUIDE

Here you'll find every stretch you'll need to do the routines outlined in this book. It can take a while to get a feel for the proper positioning and alignment of a stretch, so don't stress if your range of motion for some of these moves is very limited. Every day, you'll get a little closer to pain-free, energized movement.

You'll see that all stretches are categorized by type (dynamic or static) as well as by the primary body part being worked. Some moves also include modifications, such as options for performing it lying down or sitting on a chair, so you can get the same benefits of the stretch but from a position that feels good for you. Before performing any of these moves, read through the directions completely. When you're ready to put them into practice, remember to do what feels comfortable, and relax!

If you are brand new to stretching, start with the beginner routine to gradually familiarize yourself with the motion patterns. If you've dabbled in stretching before but aren't sure how to dive back in, start with the body parts that feel stiffest. Maybe your hips have felt tightly wound lately or your calves have been tensing up after long walks. Focus on these areas. Whatever stretching routine you decide to begin with, be patient with yourself. The very first time you lean into a calf stretch or arch into cat-cow you may feel a million miles from your mobility goals, but stick with it. With regular practice, you'll see encouraging changes in no time.

Static Stretches

Remember, static stretches are all about slow, gradual movements. Take your time as you ease into these stretches. Be sure to read the "Where You Should Feel It" notes so you can get a clear idea of how deep you need to go in each pose.

ARMS
Biceps Stretch

GOOD FOR
Shoulder pain

HOW TO DO IT
Starting Position: Standing

1. Begin standing so that the right side of your body is facing a wall. Place your right hand on the wall and adjust your footing so that you can maintain a straight arm.

2. Keeping your hand on the wall, gently rotate your body to the left so that you are facing away from your right arm and the wall. Only go until you feel a stretch in your biceps (upper arm) or your shoulder/chest area.

3. Hold for 20 to 30 seconds. Repeat 2 or 3 times on each side.

WHERE YOU SHOULD FEEL IT
Along the top and front of the upper arm, where the biceps muscles are located, or at the top of the shoulder where the tendon inserts. You may also feel a pec or chest stretch at the same time.

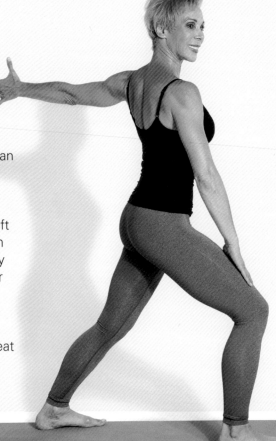

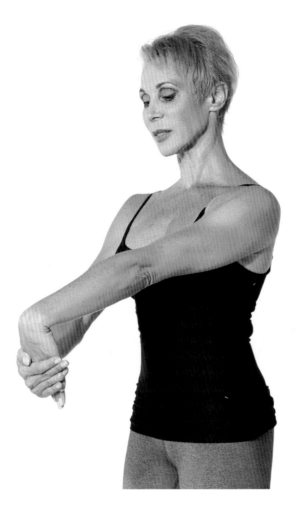

Wrist Stretch

GOOD FOR
Sitting all day
Forearms

HOW TO DO IT
Starting Position: Sitting or Standing

1. Extend your right arm in front of you with the elbow straight and palm and wrist bent so that your fingers are pointed toward the floor.

2. Use your left hand to apply gentle pressure to the top of your right hand.

3. Hold for 20 to 30 seconds. Repeat 3 times on each side.

WHERE YOU SHOULD FEEL IT
In the top of your forearm muscles.

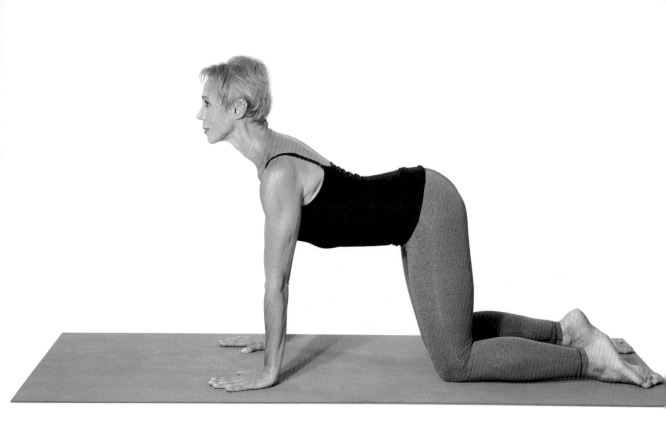

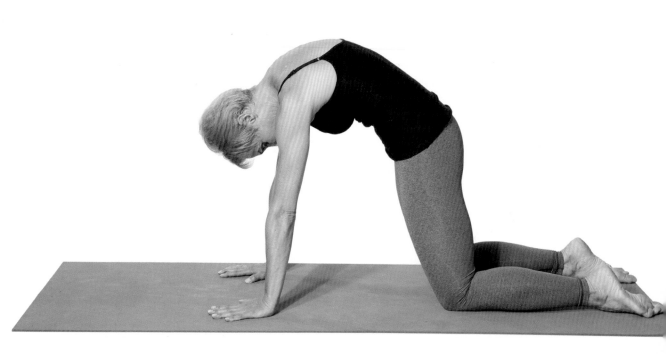

BACK
Cat-Camel

GOOD FOR
Lower back pain
Upper back pain
Shoulder pain
Beginners
Relaxation

TIP
Use this move to gently warm the whole spine and restore circulation to tight back muscles.

HOW TO DO IT
Starting Position:
Hands and Knees

1. Begin on the floor on your hands and knees with your spine in a neutral position. As you inhale, arch your back by dropping your belly button toward the floor and look up toward the ceiling. Hold.

2. Exhale as you round your back up toward the ceiling like an angry cat, lower your head, and drop your shoulders.

3. Move between these two positions gently and slowly for 5 to 8 repetitions.

WHERE YOU SHOULD FEEL IT
You should feel small movements in your spine, which can be stiff in places that are more restricted. You may also feel some muscles activating and relaxing in and around the shoulder blades.

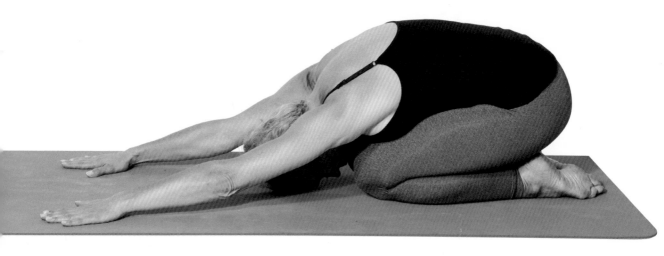

Child's Pose

GOOD FOR
Shoulder pain
Relaxation

HOW TO DO IT
Starting Position: Hands and Knees

1. Begin on your hands and knees, with your hands directly under your shoulders and knees under your hips.

2. Walk your arms out in front of you, placing your palms flat on the floor. Slowly sit your hips back toward your heels, dropping your head and chest downward as your arms extend farther in front of you. If this stretch is too much, place a pillow under your belly to prop yourself up a bit and lessen the stretch of the lower back muscles.

3. Hold for 20 to 30 seconds.

WHERE YOU SHOULD FEEL IT
In your shoulders, butt, and through the length of your spine.

Cobra Stretch

GOOD FOR
Posture
Energy
Shoulder pain

HOW TO DO IT
Starting Position: Lying Down

1. Begin by lying on your stomach with your palms face-down by your shoulders.

2. Keeping your pelvis connected with the floor, press yourself up onto your hands so that your arms straighten, your lower back is arched, and your abdomen is stretched. Look up toward the ceiling as you do so. Lift your chest and pull your shoulders back as you ground your legs. Inhale here. Hold for 20 to 30 seconds. Repeat 2 or 3 times.

WHERE YOU SHOULD FEEL IT
In your abdomen, chest, and shoulders. Avoid lower back pain by tucking your pelvis so your pubic bone comes toward the floor, and modify by going up onto only your forearms (not straight arms) if you feel any pain in your lower back.

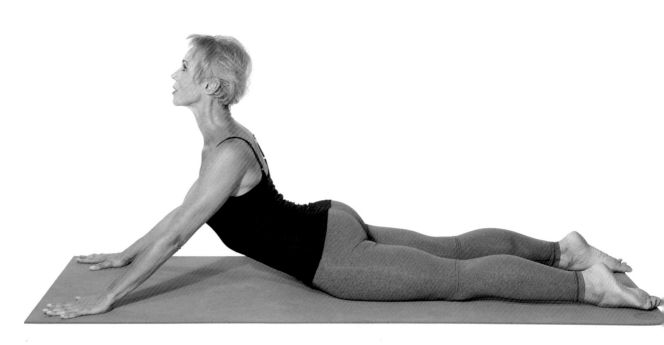

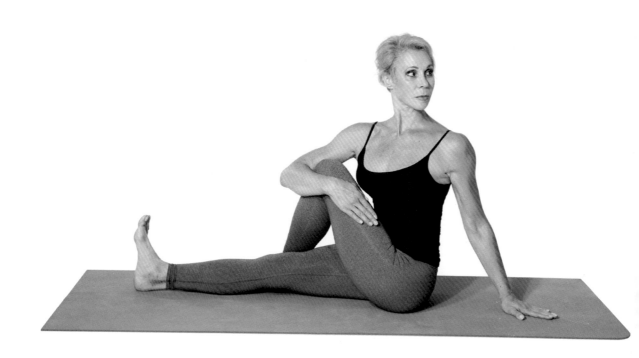

Cross-Body Knee to Chest Stretch

GOOD FOR
Hip pain

HOW TO DO IT
Starting Position: Sitting

1. Sit on the ground with your legs straight out in front of you. Bend your right leg and cross it over your left.

2. Gently hug your right knee to your chest.

3. Hold for 20 to 30 seconds. Repeat 2 or 3 times on each side.

WHERE YOU SHOULD FEEL IT
In your outer hip or buttock area of the leg that is bent.

Lower Trunk Rotation

GOOD FOR
Lower back pain
Relaxation
65+

HOW TO DO IT
Starting Position: Lying Down

1. Begin lying on your back with knees bent and arms by your side or out to the sides like the letter "T" to stabilize.

2. While keeping your upper back and shoulders on the floor, slowly allow your knees to drift all the way to the right side until you feel a ger twist and stretch in your lower back area. Try keeping your knees glued together as you do this.

3. After a few seconds, pick up your knees and allow them to fall to the left side, all while keeping knees together and shoulder blades down. Gently continue to rock side to side, allowing a few seconds of stretch as you reach the end point on each side. Repeat for 5 twists to each side.

WHERE YOU SHOULD FEEL IT
You should feel a gentle rotation and stretch in the lower back and hip area and possibly a slight stretch in your side or midback.

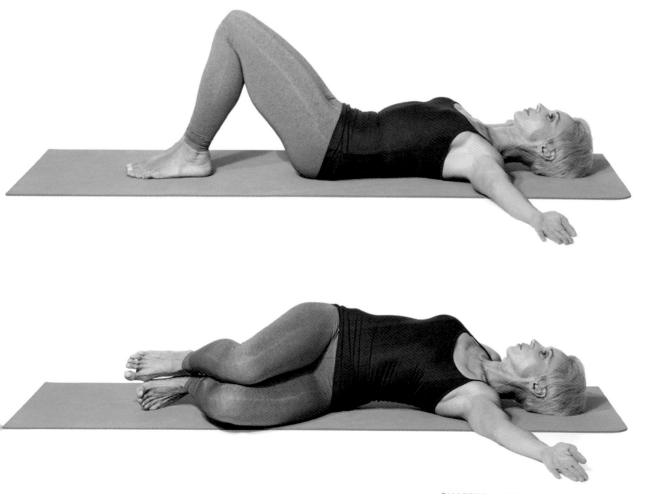

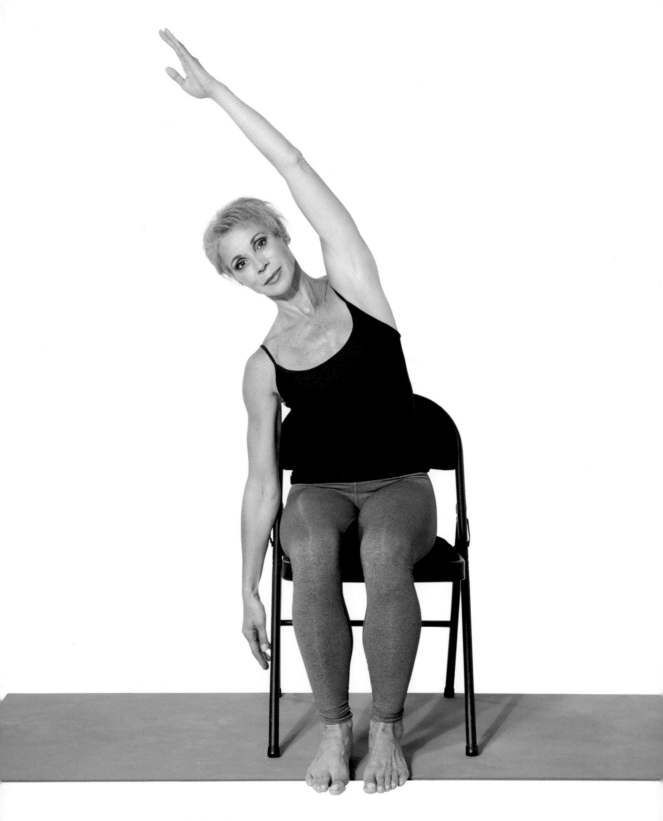

Overhead Reach with Mini Side Bend

GOOD FOR
Quick sitting stretch

HOW TO DO IT
Starting Position: Sitting

1. Begin seated in a chair with your feet firmly planted on the ground, hips square, and your back a couple inches away from the back of your chair.

2. Place your right hand on the right side of the chair and sit up tall as you reach your left arm up and over your head to the right, allowing the space between your left ribcage and pelvis to expand. Hold here for 20 seconds and breathe into your left side.

3. Return to center and repeat with your right arm. Perform 3 of these stretches on each side, slowly alternating from one side to the other, lengthening and reaching through each arm as you go.

WHERE YOU SHOULD FEEL IT
You should feel this stretch in the space between your ribs and your pelvis (at the side of your abdomen), as well as in the shoulder of the arm reaching up.

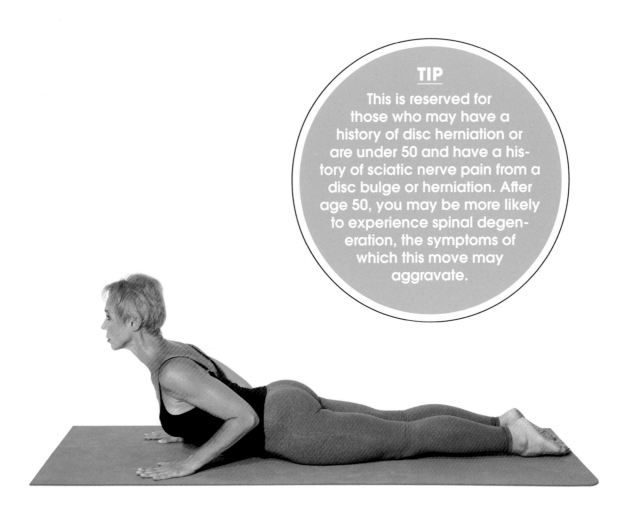

Prone Press-Up Stretch

GOOD FOR
Sciatic nerve pain

HOW TO DO IT
Starting Position: Lying Down

1. While lying flat on your stomach, place your hands on the floor near your shoulders.

2. Gently press up onto your hands, straightening your arms as much as you are comfortable doing. Allow your back to arch while relaxing your back muscles.

3. Hold for 1 to 2 seconds, then lower yourself back to the floor. Repeat 8 to 10 times, 2 or 3 times per day or as symptoms persist.

WHERE YOU SHOULD FEEL IT
In your lower back and the front of your abdomen.

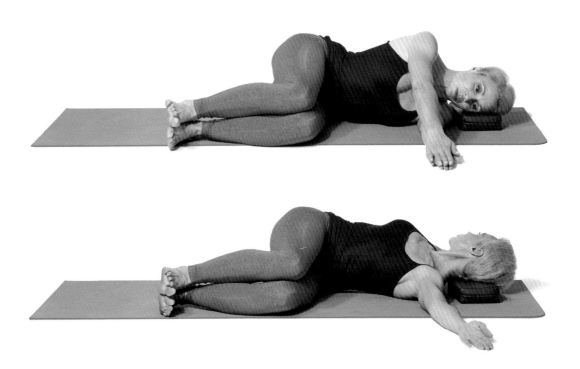

Side-Lying Thoracic Rotation

GOOD FOR
40+
65+
Flexibility
Arthritis

HOW TO DO IT
Starting Position: Lying Down

1. Using a cushion to support your head, lie on your right side with your hands and arms outstretched (palms facing each other) and knees bent.

2. While keeping your knees and hips facing forward, begin by lifting your left arm up toward the ceiling and continuing to let it fall open until your head and eyes are facing the left. Allow your spine to rotate and your pecs to stretch and open as you take a couple breaths in this twisted, open position.

3. Return to the starting position with your head facing forward, arms outstretched in front of you, and your palms touching. Repeat 8 times on each side.

WHERE YOU SHOULD FEEL IT
In your upper back. If you feel it in your lower back, try bringing your knees closer to your chest.

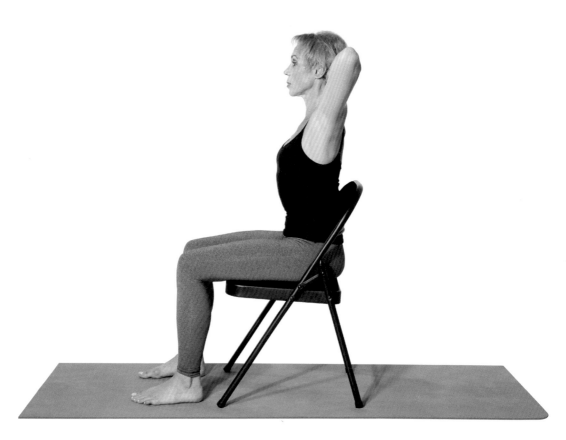

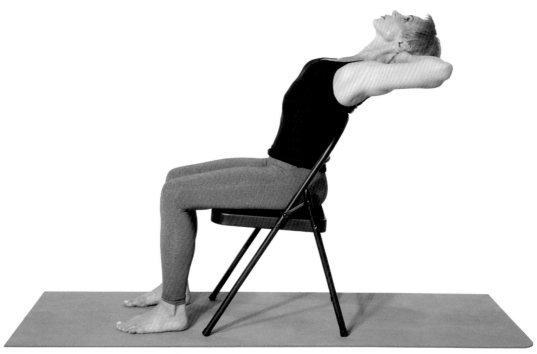

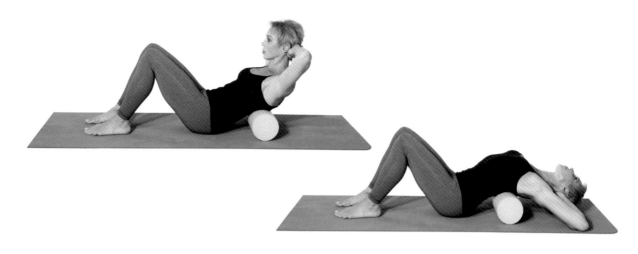

Thoracic Extension Stretch

GOOD FOR
Posture
Upper back pain

HOW TO DO IT
Starting Position: Sitting

1. Begin seated in a chair with your feet firmly planted on the ground, hips square.

2. Clasp your hands behind your head and gently arch your upper back over the back of the chair. Take a deep breath. Hold the stretch for 10 seconds then return to the starting position. Repeat 4 to 6 times.

Starting Position: Lying Down

1. Lying on the ground on your back, place a foam roller under your upper back. Place your hands behind your head to support your neck.

2. Keeping your hands behind your head, gently let your head fall back over the foam roller, allowing your upper back to extend, section by section.

3. Once your back is fully extended, gently return to the starting position. That's 1 extension. Repeat 2 extensions there then adjust the foam roller so that it is slightly higher or lower on your upper back and roll it out for 2 extensions. Follow this pattern for a total of 3 or 4 sections of your upper back.

WHERE YOU SHOULD FEEL IT
At each inflection point in your back as you arch over the chair or foam roller. You may also feel it in your chest.

CHEST
Pec Stretch

GOOD FOR
Upper back pain
Neck pain
Shoulder pain
Quick standing stretch
40+
Beginners
Flexibility
Relaxation
Posture

HOW TO DO IT
Starting Position: Standing

1. With a towel or strap in your right hand, stand straight with your feet hip-width apart, arms at your sides.

2. Move your arms straight back behind you, grabbing on to the towel with your left hand so that it is taut between your arms. If you don't have a towel, simply clasp your hands behind you.

3. Gently lift the towel up behind you. Hold for 15 to 30 seconds then lower back down. Repeat 2 or 3 times.

Starting Position: Lying Down

1. Keeping your knees bent and feet flat on the ground, lie on a foam roller so that the roller lines up with the back of your head down to your tailbone.

2. Bring your palms together in front of your chest. Slowly open your arms out to the side like the letter "T," allowing your hands to fall to the ground. Let gravity and breathwork help increase the stretch.

3. Hold for 30 seconds, then bring your hands back to center. Repeat 3 times.

WHERE YOU SHOULD FEEL IT
In your chest.

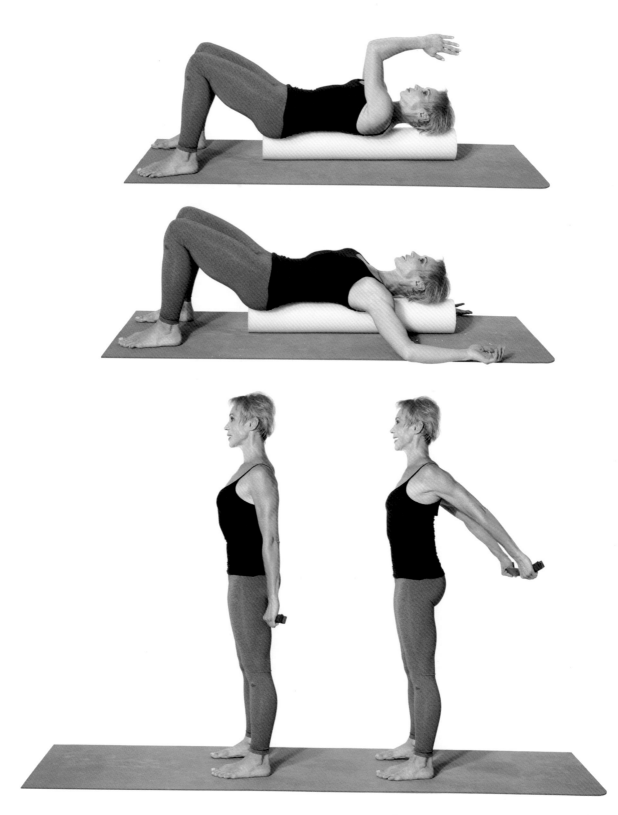

HIPS
Butterfly Stretch

GOOD FOR
Hip pain
Flexibility

HOW TO DO IT
Starting Position: Sitting

1. Sit on the floor so that your knees are bent open to opposite sides and the soles of your feet are facing each other.

2. Clasp both feet with your hands and slowly bend forward. For an extra stretch, allow your elbows to rest on your knees and apply a little pressure during the stretch.

3. Hold for 20 to 30 seconds, then return to sitting up straight. Repeat 2 to 3 times.

WHERE YOU SHOULD FEEL IT
In your groin along your inner thigh.

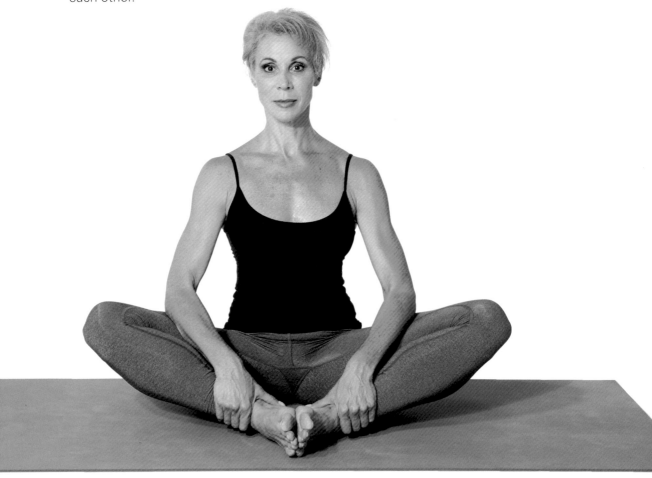

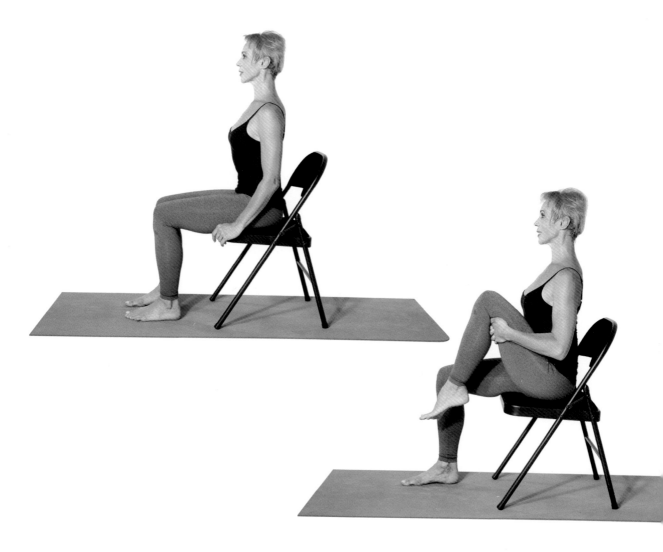

Knee to Chest Stretch

GOOD FOR
Hip pain
Relaxation

HOW TO DO IT
Starting Position: Sitting

1. Sit up straight in a chair with both feet planted on the ground.

2. Raise your right knee to your chest, clasping your hands around the front of your knee or the back of your thigh.

3. Hug your leg for 30 seconds, then lower it back to the ground. Repeat on the left side, performing 2 or 3 reps per side.

WHERE YOU SHOULD FEEL IT
In your hips and lower back.

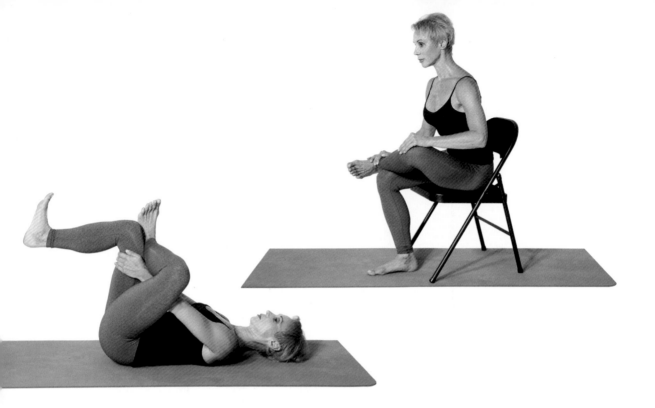

Figure Four Stretch

GOOD FOR
Hip pain
40+
Flexibility
Arthritis

HOW TO DO IT
Starting Position: Lying Down

1. Lie on your back with both knees bent.

2. Cross your right ankle over your left knee so that your ankle rests on top of your knee. Grab behind your left thigh and pull that knee in toward your chest until you feel a pull or stretch in your right hip.

3. Hold for 20 to 30 seconds, then lower your leg back down. Repeat 2 or 3 times on each side.

Starting Position: Sitting

1. Sit up straight in a chair with both feet planted on the ground.

2. Cross your right ankle over your left knee so that your ankle rests over the top of your knee. Lean forward.

3. Hold for 20 to 30 seconds, then sit up straight again. Repeat 2 or 3 times.

WHERE YOU SHOULD FEEL IT
In the hip of the leg that's on top of your knee.

Double Knee to Chest Stretch

GOOD FOR
Hip pain
Arthritis
65+

HOW TO DO IT
Starting Position: Lying Down

1. Begin by lying on your back with your knees bent, feet flat on the floor, and arms at your sides.

2. With your hands either behind your thighs or slightly below your kneecaps, slowly bring both knees toward your chest.

3. Hold here for 20 to 30 seconds. Try rocking your hips side to side and up and down to help massage your lower back. Return to starting position. Repeat 2 or 3 times.

WHERE YOU SHOULD FEEL IT
In your lower back as you bring your knees to your chest.

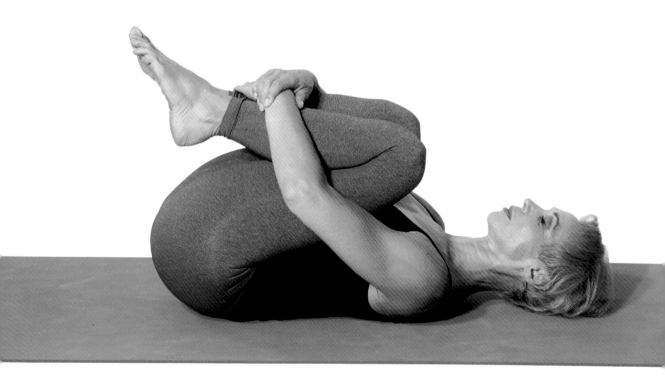

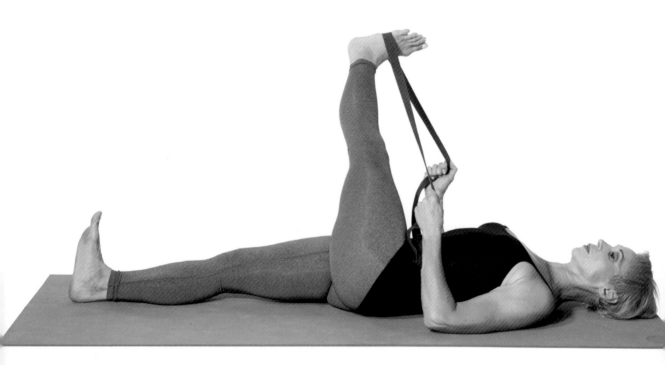

IT Band "Stretch"

GOOD FOR
Knee pain

HOW TO DO IT
Starting Position: Lying Down

1. Start lying on your back with your right leg in a hamstring stretch with a strap (p. 108).

2. Draw your right leg diagonally across your body while it is elevated to increase the stretch along the outer hip and thigh.

3. Hold it there for 20 to 30 seconds, then lower your leg and release the strap so that you are lying flat on the ground. Repeat 2 or 3 times on each side.

WHERE YOU SHOULD FEEL IT
Along your outer hip and thigh.

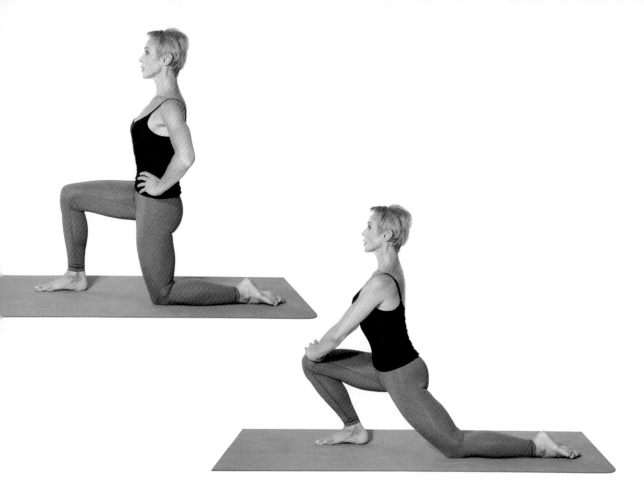

Kneeling Lunge Stretch with Bent Knee

GOOD FOR
Hip pain

HOW TO DO IT
Starting Position: Kneeling

1. Place a towel on the ground and kneel on it with both knees.

2. Step your right leg forward so that it is bent at about a 90-degree angle. Rest your hands on the front of your right thigh.

3. With your spine upright, tuck your tailbone and lean forward into your right leg until you feel a stretch along the front of your left hip.

4. Hold for 5 breaths, then repeat with your left leg forward.

WHERE YOU SHOULD FEEL IT
In the front of the hip of the leg that is kneeling.

Lunge Stretch with Overhead Reach

GOOD FOR
Hip pain
Walkers
Flexibility

HOW TO DO IT
Starting Position: Standing

1. With your hands on your hips, stagger your legs so your right foot is in front of your left. Inch your left foot backward so that your right knee begins to bend and your left leg is straight. Make sure your right knee doesn't go past your toes and both heels stay on the ground.

2. Reach your left arm up toward the ceiling, then over the top of your body toward the right. Take the arch out of your lower back by tucking your tailbone under. Lean into the stretch, breathing into the tightest area and sinking deeper into the stretch as you exhale.

3. Hold for 20 to 30 seconds, then return to the starting lunge position. Repeat 2 or 3 times on each side.

WHERE YOU SHOULD FEEL IT
In the front of your hip and deep in your lower abdomen and pelvis area. You may even feel it in the side of your body as you reach your arm up and over.

Hip Stretch
Off Elevated Surface

GOOD FOR
Lower back pain
Hip pain
40+
Posture

HOW TO DO IT
Starting Position: Lying Down

1. Begin lying on your back on an elevated surface, such as a firm bed, with your butt at the edge. Your legs should be bent and hanging off the edge.

2. Scoot to the right side of the bed so that the right side of your pelvis can hang off the side edge freely.

3. Grab your left knee slightly below your kneecap and hug it toward your chest. Try not to let your back arch. Allow your right leg to hang off of the edge of the surface, reaching toward the floor, and let gravity open up your right hip. With every exhale, allow yourself to sink deeper into the stretch. Hold for 30 seconds, then place your left leg back on the ground. Repeat 2 or 3 times on each side.

WHERE YOU SHOULD FEEL IT
This stretch is both a healing stretch and a somewhat diagnostic stretch, meaning it can help highlight where you feel the most tension. You may feel the stretch in the front of the thigh of the leg hanging off the edge. You may also feel a stretch along the outer knee of this same leg as well as deep in the lower abdomen/pelvis area.

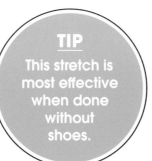

TIP
This stretch is most effective when done without shoes.

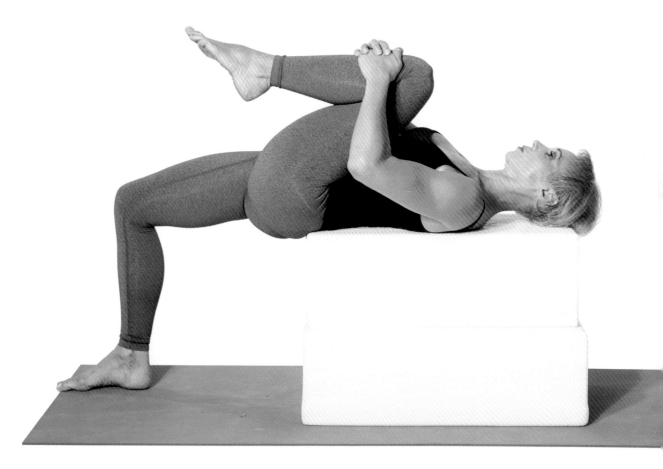

LEGS & LOWER BODY
Big Toe Stretch

GOOD FOR
Heel pain

HOW TO DO IT
Starting Position: Standing

1. Stand facing a wall or a yoga block, and stagger your legs so your right foot is in front of your left. Place your palms flat against the wall.

2. Move your right foot so that your big toe is up against the wall but your heel and the rest of your foot remain on the floor.

3. Lean into the stretch so that your big toe is extended upward (perpendicular to the floor).

4. Hold for 20 seconds, then release your big toe so it is back on the ground. Repeat 2 or 3 times on each side.

WHERE YOU SHOULD FEEL IT
Anywhere along the bottom of your big toe or across the medial (or inner) arch of your foot and possibly even into your lower leg.

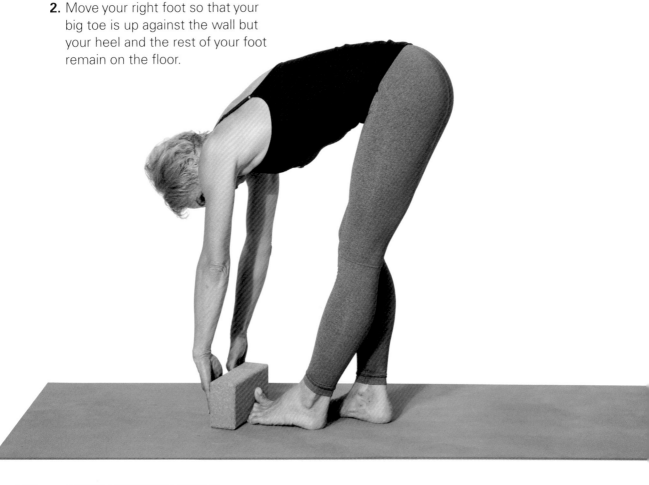

Calf Stretch

GOOD FOR
Knee pain
Heel pain
Quick standing stretch
Hikers
Walkers
Beginners
Arthritis

HOW TO DO IT
Starting Position: Standing

1. Stand facing a wall at about arm's length. Stagger your left leg slightly in front of your right.

2. Place your hands on the wall in front of you, slightly bending your left leg and pressing your right heel down. You may need to spread your feet more so that you start to feel a stretch in your right leg. Keep both heels in contact with the floor.

3. Hold for 30 seconds, then switch legs. Repeat 2 times on each side.

WHERE YOU SHOULD FEEL IT
In the calf of the back leg. If you don't, try shifting your weight to your front foot a little more.

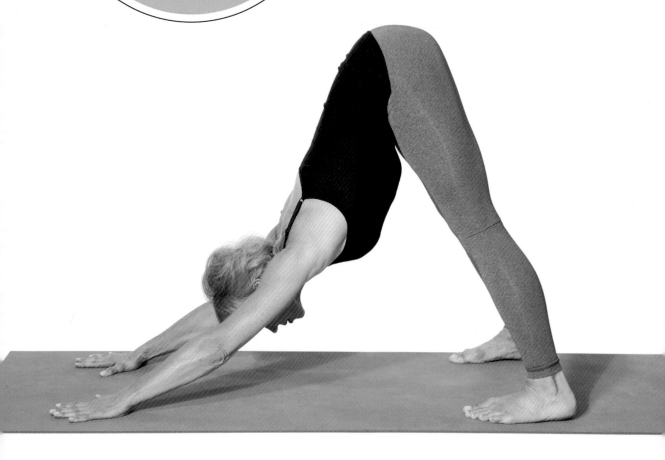

Downward Dog

GOOD FOR
Beginners

HOW TO DO IT
Starting Position: Hands and Knees

1. Begin on the floor on your hands and knees. Make sure your hands are about shoulder-width apart and your fingers and toes are pointed forward.

2. Lift up off your knees so you are putting your weight through your hands and feet only.

3. Lift your butt up toward the ceiling and gently straighten your knees, adjusting the spacing of your hands and feet as needed so that you can keep your heels down on the floor.

4. Press through your palms and firm the outer arms as you sink into this stretch. Hold for up to 1 minute, then return to your hands and knees. If it feels good, you can pedal your feet, bending one knee at a time to achieve a deeper stretch in the calves. Repeat 3 times.

WHERE YOU SHOULD FEEL IT
In the back of your legs—your hamstrings and calves—and heels. You may also feel some muscle activation and possibly a stretching in your shoulder area.

Hamstring Stretch

GOOD FOR
Lower back pain
Knee pain
Heel pain
Walkers
40+
65+
Beginners
Flexibility
Arthritis

HOW TO DO IT
Starting Position: Lying Down

1. Lie flat on your back with both legs outstretched.

2. Using a stretching strap, yoga strap, or towel, wrap a loop around your right foot.

3. Maintaining a good grip on the strap with both hands, slowly use your arms to elevate your leg straight up toward the ceiling. Do not let your knee bend. Go until you feel a pull in the back of your thigh but no sharp pain.

4. Hold this position for 30 seconds, then slowly lower your leg back down. Repeat 3 or 4 times on each side.

Starting Position: Standing

1. Begin standing tall, with feet hip-width apart and legs straight.

2. Keeping your legs straight, slowly roll down toward the floor beginning with your head, followed by your neck, your shoulders, and each vertebra of your spine one at a time. Lower until your hands are reaching toward the floor.

3. Let yourself hang there for 20 to 30 seconds before slowly rolling back up. Repeat 3 or 4 times.

Starting Position: Sitting

1. Sit on the ground with your legs straight out in front of you.

2. Slowly bend forward and reach your arms toward your toes, keeping your knees straight or slightly bent. Grab your lower legs or ankles to help maintain the position.

3. Hold for 20 to 30 seconds, then return to the starting position. Repeat 3 times.

WHERE YOU SHOULD FEEL IT
In the lying-down position, you should feel a pull in the back of the thigh that is being worked. In the standing and seated positions, you should feel a pull in the back of your hips and the thighs of both legs.

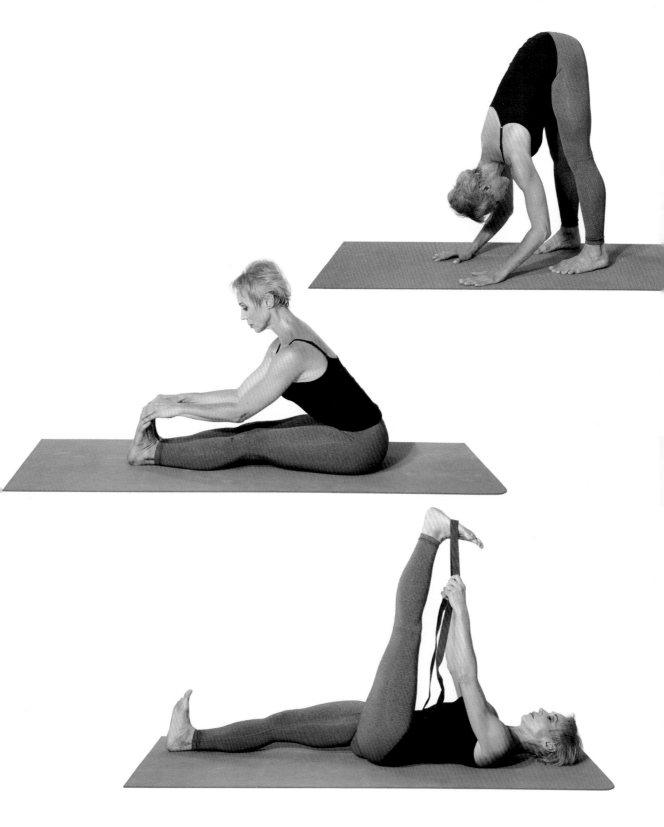

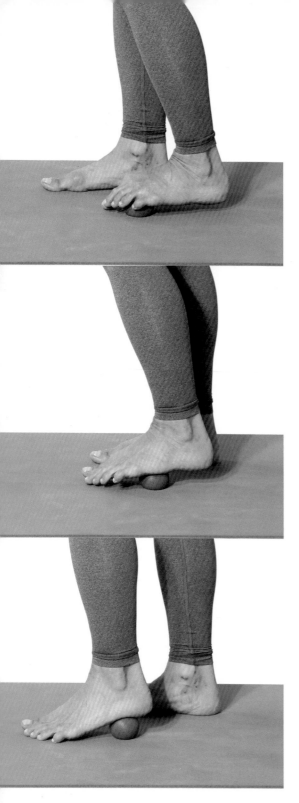

Plantar Fascia Rollout

GOOD FOR
Standing all day

HOW TO DO IT
Starting Position: Sitting or Standing

1. Place a lacrosse or tennis ball under your foot and simply roll your foot over the ball, first longitudinally (heel to toes), then in horizontal sections beginning at the base of the heel and moving little by little up toward the toes.

2. Repeat for a few minutes then switch sides.

WHERE YOU SHOULD FEEL IT
In the bottom of your foot in the band of tissue between your toes and heel. It may be particularly sensitive closer to the heel and the inner part of the arch of your foot.

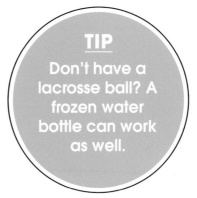

TIP
Don't have a lacrosse ball? A frozen water bottle can work as well.

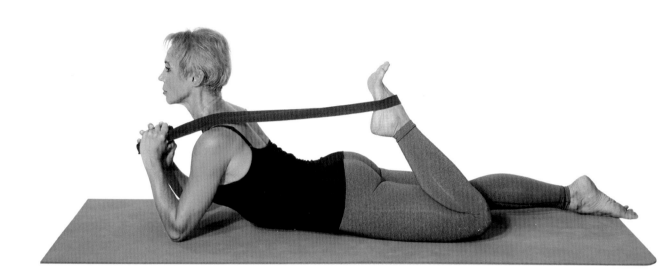

Prone Quad Stretch

GOOD FOR
Tight quads

HOW TO DO IT
Starting Position: Lying Down

1. While lying on your stomach, bend your right leg toward your butt and loop a stretching strap or towel around your right foot.

2. Gently pull the strap or towel so your right foot moves toward your butt. Be sure not to fight the pull. Keep your right leg relaxed.

3. Hold for 30 seconds, then release your leg. Repeat 2 or 3 times on each side.

WHERE YOU SHOULD FEEL IT
In the front of the thigh and hip of the side you are stretching. If you feel it in your lower back, try tucking your pelvis so your pubic bone moves toward the floor instead of letting your back arch. You can also lighten up on the pull of the strap.

Soleus Stretch

GOOD FOR
Heel pain

HOW TO DO IT
Starting Position: Standing

1. Start like you are doing a calf stretch (p. 105). Stand facing a wall at about arm's length. Stagger your left leg slightly in front of your right.

2. Place your hands on the wall in front of you, slightly bending your left leg and pressing your right heel down.

3. Bend your right leg slightly.

4. Hold 30 seconds for 2 or 3 repetitions on each side.

WHERE YOU SHOULD FEEL IT
This stretch will be felt a little lower down than the calf stretch. You'll likely feel it in the lower part of the lower leg and into the Achilles tendon area. It's a slightly deeper stretch than the straight knee calf stretch, which can usually be felt more in the superficial bulging muscle belly area (a.k.a. the thickest part of your muscle).

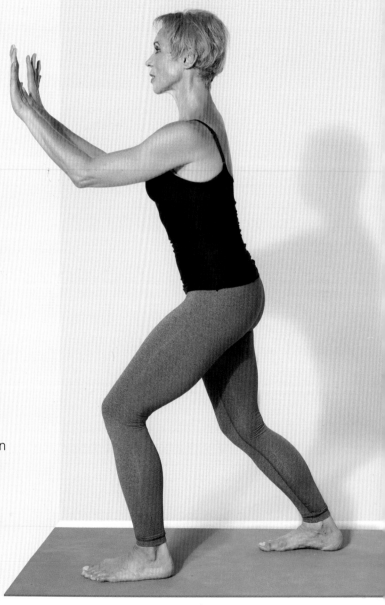

Quad Stretch

GOOD FOR
Knee pain

HOW TO DO IT
Starting Position: Standing

1. Stand with your feet about hip-width apart.

2. Holding onto a wall or chair for balance with your left hand, bring your right foot to your right hand by bending your right leg back toward your butt.

3. Gently pull your right foot closer toward your butt without arching your back. Slightly tuck your tailbone under for a deeper stretch.

4. Hold for 20 to 30 seconds, then lower your foot to the ground. Repeat 3 or 4 times on each side.

WHERE YOU SHOULD FEEL IT
Along the front of your thigh and possibly at the knee and front of the hip.

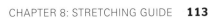

NECK
Chin Tucks

GOOD FOR
Neck pain

HOW TO DO IT
Starting Position: Lying Down

1. Lie on the ground with your knees bent and arms at your side.

2. Gently tuck your chin down, and contract the muscles in your neck by pushing your head back toward the floor as if you are making a double chin.

3. Hold for 10 seconds, then release. Repeat 6 to 8 times.

WHERE YOU SHOULD FEEL IT
At the base of your skull where your neck meets your head.

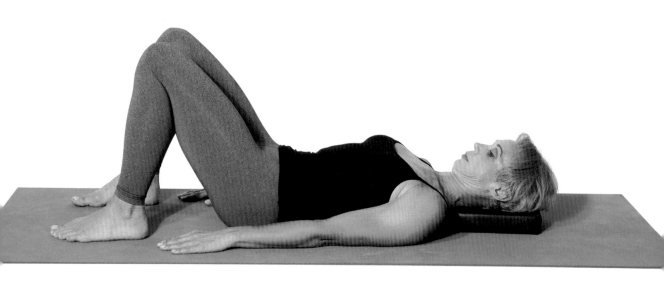

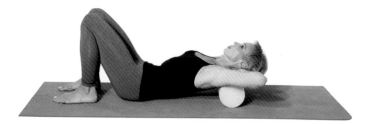

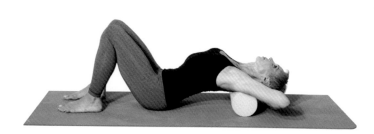

Neck Extension over Foam Roller

GOOD FOR
Neck pain

HOW TO DO IT
Starting Position: Lying Down

1. Begin lying on the ground with your hands behind your head and your neck resting over a foam roller. Bend your knees.

2. Keeping your head supported with your hands and your hips on the ground, gently rock your neck backward like you are looking up. Continue for 10 to 20 seconds.

3. Turn your head slightly to the right. While looking to the right, gently move your neck side to side to release any restrictions in the muscles along the side of your neck. Continue for 10 to 20 seconds, then return to the starting position. Repeat 2 or 3 times on each side.

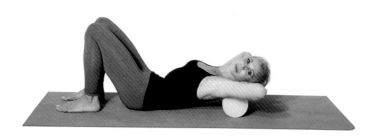

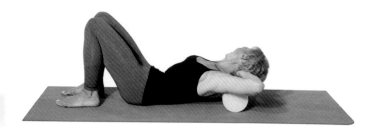

WHERE YOU SHOULD FEEL IT
In the muscles at the back of your neck and slightly to the sides of them.

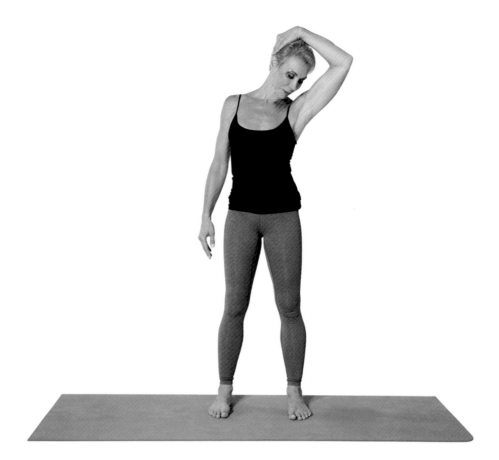

Levator Scap Stretch

GOOD FOR
Neck pain

HOW TO DO IT
Starting Position: Sitting or Standing

1. Put your right hand on the back of your head, and gently guide your head so it is tilted down and to the right, like you are going to smell your right armpit.

2. Hold for 20 to 30 seconds, then lift your head up. Repeat 2 or 3 times on each side.

WHERE YOU SHOULD FEEL IT
At the base of your neck on the side you are turning away from. You may also feel a stretch along the taut muscles that lead to the top of your shoulder.

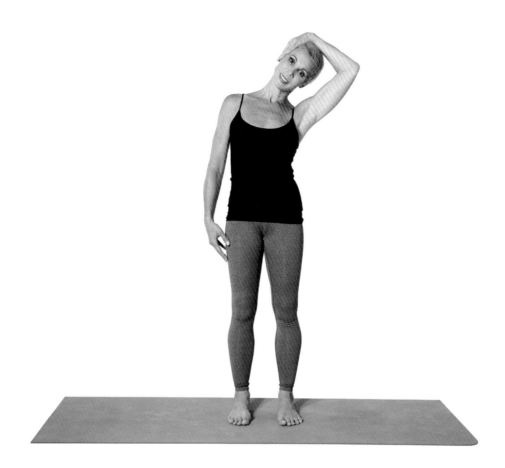

Upper Trap Stretch

GOOD FOR
Upper back pain
Neck pain

HOW TO DO IT
Starting Position: Sitting or Standing

1. Begin sitting or standing with your head centered and neck long.

2. Raise your right hand up and over your head, and place it on the left side of your head.

3. Applying gentle pressure with your hand, lower your right ear to your right shoulder. Do not rotate your head. Keep it in the same plane of movement, as if there is a pane of glass in front and behind your head.

4. Hold for 20 to 30 seconds, then return to the starting position. Repeat 3 or 4 times on each side.

WHERE YOU SHOULD FEEL IT
In the muscle between your neck and your shoulder on the side that is being elongated (so when you're bending toward the right, you should feel the stretch on your left).

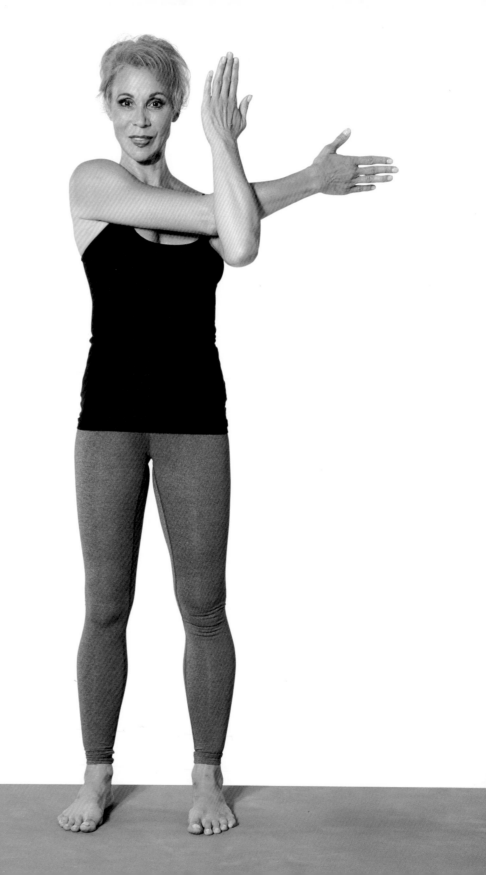

SHOULDERS

Arm Across Chest Stretch

GOOD FOR
Shoulder pain

HOW TO DO IT
Starting Position: Standing

1. Stand with your feet about hip-width apart.

2. Raise your left arm straight in front of you. Use your right arm to grab your left arm slightly above your elbow, then gently pull your left arm straight across your body.

3. Hold for 20 seconds, then release. Repeat 3 times on each side.

WHERE YOU SHOULD FEEL IT
In the shoulder of the arm being pulled across your chest.

Dynamic Stretches

As you now know, dynamic stretches are done while moving, gradually opening you to a greater range of motion. These quick movements are used to promote blood flow and elongate the muscles that are going to be used in a given activity. Because you are functioning through a range of motion instead of the same position the whole time, there isn't just one place you should feel these stretches. Instead, simply stay alert for any pain (pain = something isn't right). Start with smaller movements, and eventually go bigger as you feel warmed up.

Arm Swings

GOOD FOR
Quick standing stretch
Energy

HOW TO DO IT
Starting Position: Standing

1. Stand with your feet about hip-width apart.

2. Begin swinging your arms forward and backward for several seconds, then in and out (like you are hugging yourself) for several seconds.

3. Continue for 30 to 60 seconds, alternating between the movements as you go.

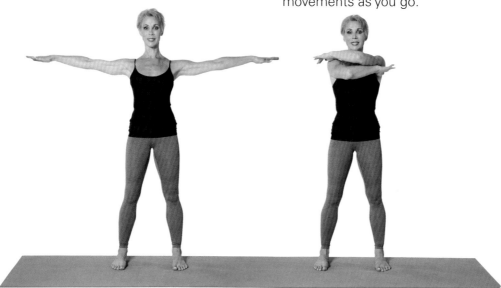

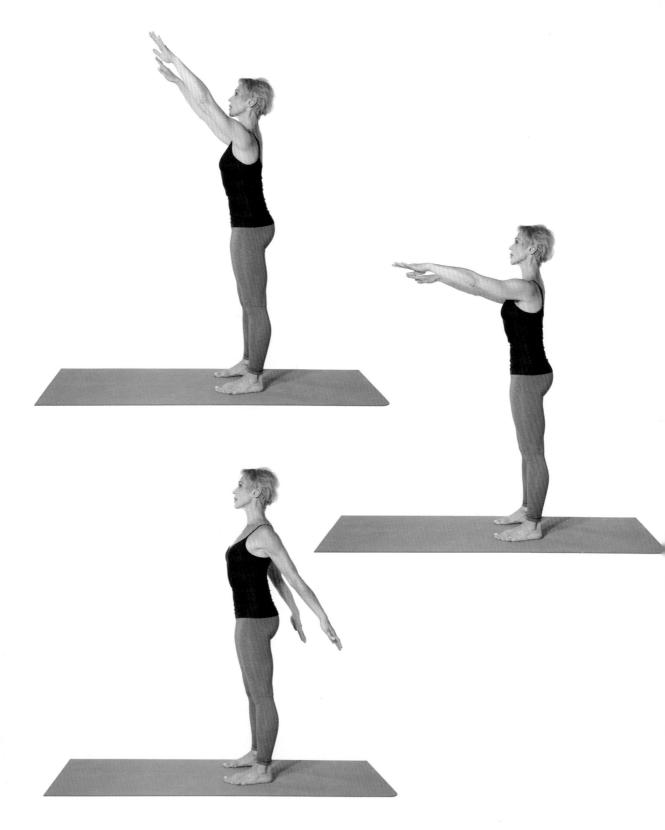

Butt Kicks

GOOD FOR
Runners
Quick walking stretch

HOW TO DO IT
Starting Position: Standing

1. Begin by jogging in place, then start kicking your heels to your butt with each step, alternating feet.

2. Continue for 30 to 60 seconds for 1 to 3 rounds.

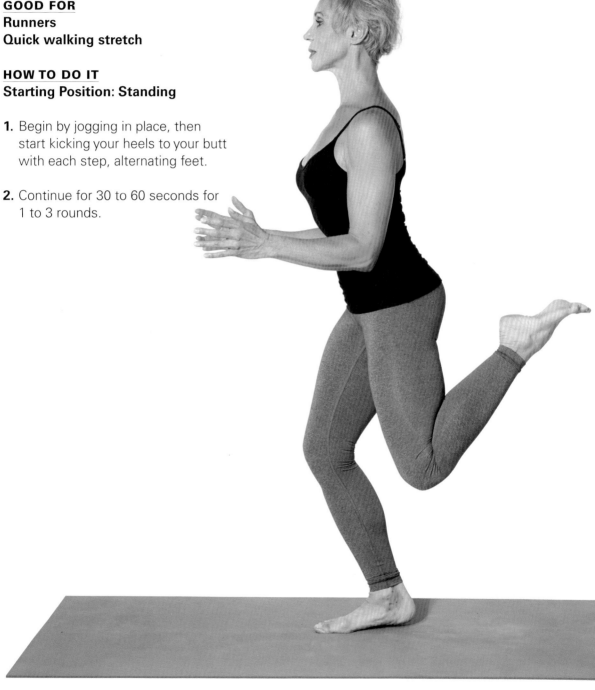

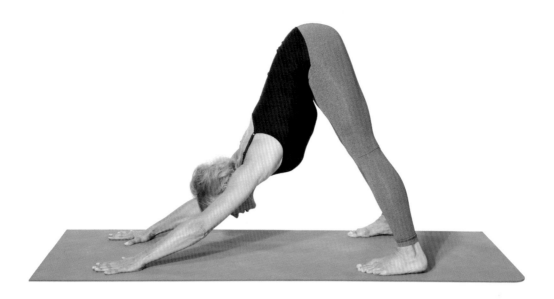

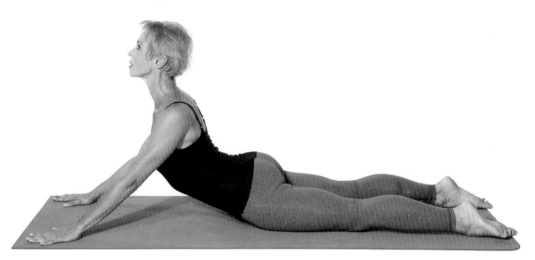

Downward Dog to Cobra

GOOD FOR
Energy

HOW TO DO IT
Starting Position: Hands and Knees

1. Begin in downward dog (p. 107) and hold for 30 to 60 seconds.

2. Then transition to cobra stretch (p. 82) by bending your arms and lowering your body to the ground, then up into cobra. Hold for 30 to 60 seconds.

3. Repeat this back-and-forth sequence 3 to 5 times to help get the blood flowing and the muscles on opposite sides of your body warmed up and lengthened.

Frankensteins

GOOD FOR
Runners

HOW TO DO IT
Starting Position: Standing

1. Swing your left leg forward, simultaneously reaching your hands out to tap your left toes (or as close as you can get).

2. Alternate between your left and right side. You will travel forward, walking like Frankenstein, as you go. Repeat for 10 reps on each side.

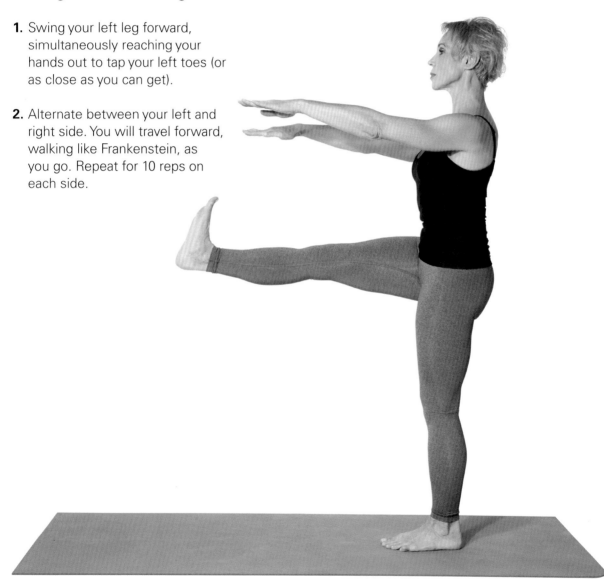

High Knees

GOOD FOR
Quick walking stretch
Runners
Energy

HOW TO DO IT
Starting Position: Standing

1. Begin hopping from one leg to the other, raising the leg that's in the air up to hip height each time. To ensure you lift each leg high enough, you can keep your arms outstretched in front of you and tap your knees to your hands as you go.

2. Continue hopping for 30 to 60 seconds.

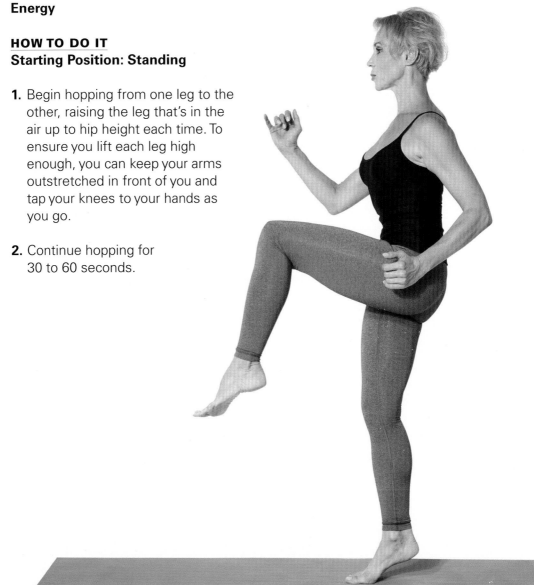

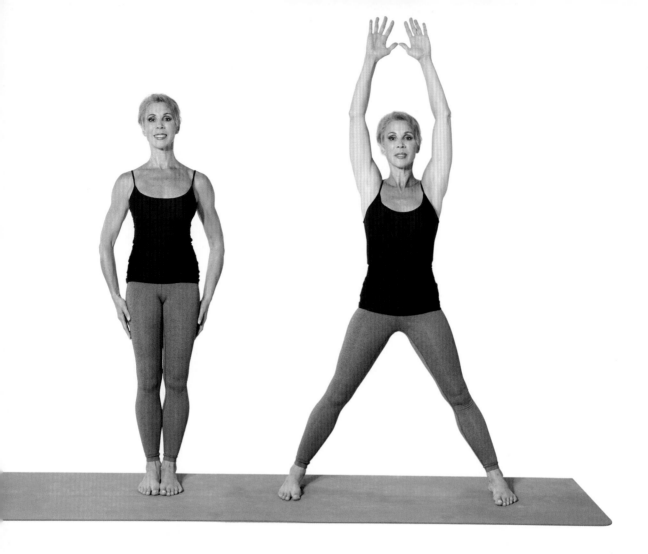

Jumping Jacks

GOOD FOR
Runners
Jumping activities/sports

HOW TO DO IT
Starting Position: Standing

1. Raise your arms overhead to about a 45-degree angle, palms facing forward. Simultaneously, jump so that your legs are a little wider than hip-width, landing with legs slightly bent.

2. Jump back to start, lowering your arms to your sides at the same time.

3. Continue for 30 to 60 seconds.

Leg Swings

GOOD FOR
Runners
Jumping sports/activities

HOW TO DO IT
Starting Position: Standing

1. Begin standing with your left side facing a wall or chair. Hold on to the wall or chair with your left hand.

2. Begin swinging your right leg forward and backward, keeping your leg straight when it's forward and leaving a slight bend in your standing leg if needed. Move your leg at a speed and to a height that feels comfortable with a slight stretch but no sharp pain.

3. Repeat 10 times or for 30 seconds on one side, then repeat on the other side.

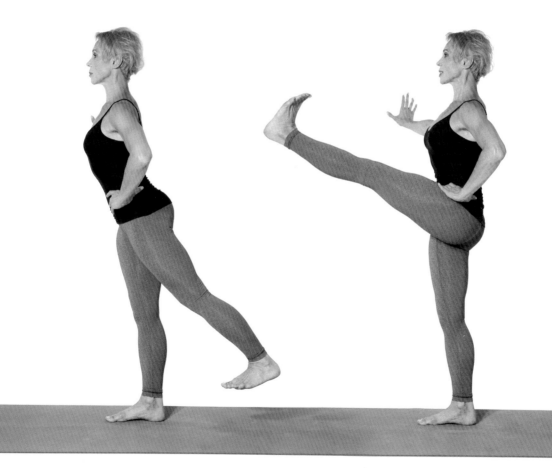

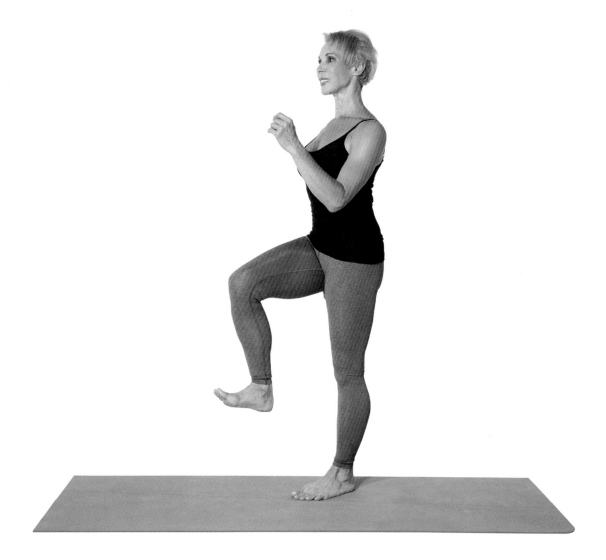

March in Place

GOOD FOR
Hikers

HOW TO DO IT
Starting Position: Standing

1. Raise your right knee to hip height, bending your right leg as you go and simultaneously raising your left arm to chest height, elbow bent.

2. Repeat on the opposite side, and continue alternating between sides without pausing for 30 to 60 seconds.

Side Shuffles

GOOD FOR
Soccer players
Runners

Starting Position: Standing

1. To shuffle right, take a few quick steps to the right using your right foot with your left foot trailing, keeping your body facing forward.

2. Shuffle to the right for about 20 to 40 feet, then reverse and shuffle to the left. Repeat for 2 or 3 rounds.

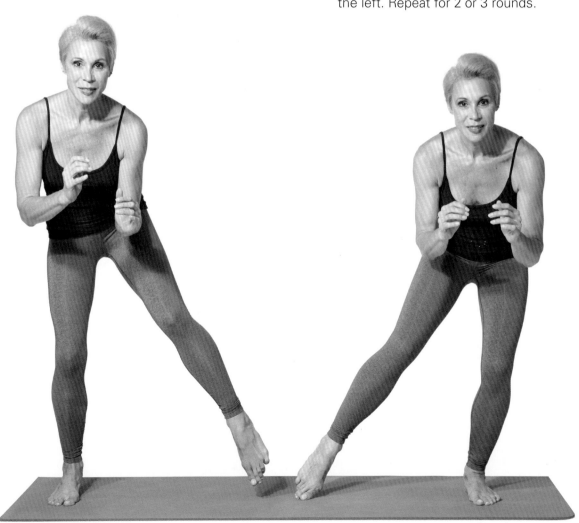

Skipping

GOOD FOR
Runners
Jumping sports/activities

HOW TO DO IT
Starting Position: Standing

1. Raise your right knee and leap up and forward, landing on your left foot. Hop forward slightly with your left leg before bringing down your right foot and repeating the pattern on your right side.

2. Alternate sides for 30 to 60 seconds, then pause. Repeat 2 or 3 times.

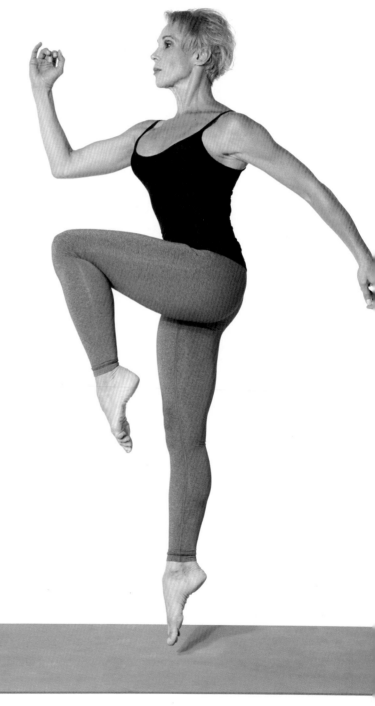

Squats

GOOD FOR
Runners
Hikers
Jumping sports/activities
HIIT workout warmup

HOW TO DO IT
Starting Position: Standing

1. Stand with your feet hip-width apart and your hands by your sides.

2. Tightening your core and glutes, sit back into your heels and push your butt back and down, lowering your body until your thighs are parallel to the ground. Look forward—not up or down—and keep your back straight and chest lifted. Make sure your heels aren't lifting off the ground and are firmly in place. Your knees and ankles shouldn't cave inward either.

3. Keeping your back upright and your core braced, push off of your heels to stand back up. Repeat for 2 or 3 sets of 10 squats with short (10- to 20-second) breaks between sets.

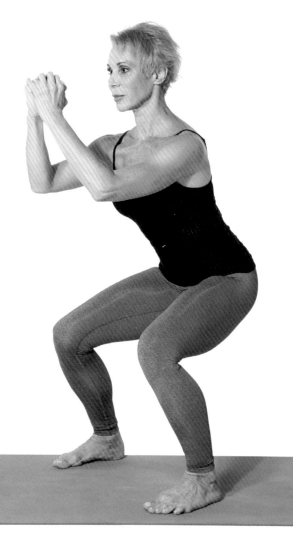

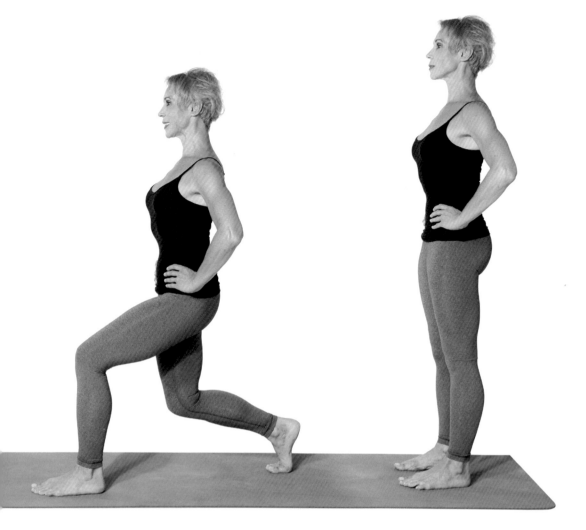

Walking Lunges

GOOD FOR
Runners
Energy

HOW TO DO IT
Starting Position: Standing

1. Begin standing with your hands on your hips or out to the side for balance.

2. Take a large, exaggerated step with your right leg and lower yourself to the ground, controlling the lowering with your right leg while using your left leg to help balance.

3. Rise back up to standing and alternate, taking the next exaggerated step with your left leg before lowering to the ground and rising back up.

4. Repeat for 60 seconds or 10 times on each side.

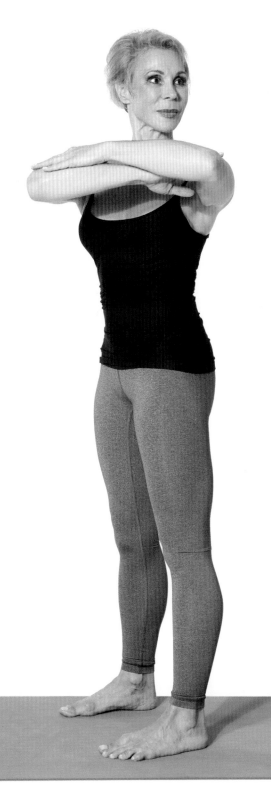

Trunk Twists

GOOD FOR
Swimmers

HOW TO DO IT
Starting Position: Standing

1. Gently twist your upper torso right to left, keeping your feet and pelvis stable but allowing your arms and shoulders to move with your torso.

2. Repeat 10 times.

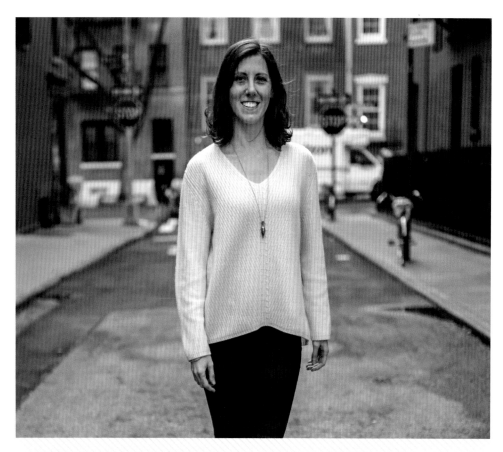

ABOUT THE EXPERT

Dr. Rachel Tavel, PT, DPT, CSCS, is a doctor of physical therapy, certified strength and conditioning specialist, and freelance writer who has helped countless patients ages 5 to 95 alleviate pain through stretching and other exercises. She earned her BA from Bowdoin College and her DPT from New York University. Rachel worked as a travel writer in South America before returning to school to become a physical therapist. She currently balances her time working as a physical therapist, helping manage and run a private practice in Manhattan, and freelance writing on the side. She is a regular contributor to *Men's Health*, *Runner's World*, and *Self* magazines, and she has been a featured expert for Sirius XM Radio's "Doctor Radio" show, as well as in multiple other health and fitness articles. You can follow her on social media at **@travelswtavel** or check out her online portfolio at **http://rtavel.journoportfolio.com**.

Thank You for Purchasing Stretch Yourself Healthy!

WE HOPE YOU ENJOYED THE GUIDE!

If you are interested in expanding your fitness library,
we have many more programs to help you reach your goals.

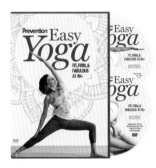
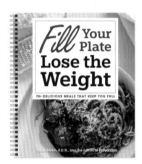
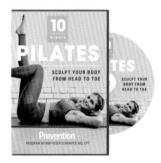